# Chiquis
# KETO

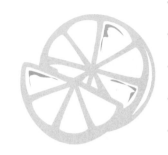

# The 21-Day Starter Kit for Taco, Tortilla, and Tequila Lovers

# Chiquis KETO

## CHIQUIS RIVERA

with **Sarah Koudouzian**

**ATRIA** PAPERBACK

New York · London · Toronto · Sydney · New Delhi

**ATRIA**
PAPERBACK

An Imprint of Simon & Schuster, Inc.
1230 Avenue of the Americas
New York, NY 10020

This publication contains the opinions and ideas of its author. It is sold with the understanding that the author and publisher are not engaged in rendering health services in the book. The reader should consult his or her own medical and health providers as appropriate before adopting any of the suggestions in this book or drawing inferences from it.

The author and publisher specifically disclaim all responsibility for any liability, loss or risk, personal or otherwise, which is incurred as a consequence, directly or indirectly, of the use and application of any of the contents of this book.

First Atria Paperback edition April 2020

**ATRIA** PAPERBACK and colophon are trademarks of Simon & Schuster, Inc.

For information about special discounts for bulk purchases,
please contact Simon & Schuster Special Sales
at 1-866-506-1949 or business@simonandschuster.com.

The Simon & Schuster Speakers Bureau can bring authors to your live event. For more
information or to book an event, contact the Simon & Schuster Speakers Bureau
at 1-866-248-3049 or visit our website at www.simonspeakers.com.

Select design graphics by Raymond Morales
Food photographs by Natalia Wrobel Katz
Lifestyle and workout photographs by Francis Bertrand

Manufactured in the United States of America

1   3   5   7   9   10   8   6   4   2

Library of Congress Cataloging-in-Publication Data

Names: Rivera, Chiquis, author. | Koudouzian, Sarah, author.
Title: Chiquis keto : the 21-day starter kit for taco, tortilla, and
tequila lovers / Chiquis Rivera with Sarah Koudouzian.
Description: First edition. | New York : Atria Paperback, 2020. | Includes index.
Identifiers: LCCN 2019057681 | ISBN 9781982133726
(paperback) | ISBN 9781982133733 (ebook)
Subjects: LCSH: Cooking, Mexican. | Ketogenic diet. | High-protein Diet—
Recipes. | Low-carbohydrate diet—Recipes. | LCGFT: Cookbooks.
Classification: LCC TX716.M4 R546 2020 | DDC 641.5972—dc23
LC record available at https://lccn.loc.gov/2019057681

ISBN 978-1-9821-3372-6
ISBN 978-1-9821-3373-3 (ebook)

# Contents

*Warning!*     vii

*Glossary*     ix

*Introduction*     xi

**ONE:** Keto . . . *¿qué?*     1

**TWO:** Keto My Way: I Don't Break the Rules, I Bend Them     11

**THREE:** The 21-Day Plan     25

**FOUR:** Chi-Keto Recipes     49

**FIVE:** The 12 Essential Exercises for a *Chingona*'s Body     161

**SIX:** Keep It Up—This Is Now *Your* Lifestyle!     171

*Acknowledgments*     177

*Index*     179

# Warning!

This is not your average keto book.

We will not be counting calories or macros.

We will not be peeing on sticks.

And we will not be beating ourselves up
if we aren't in a state of ketosis 24/7.

This is keto done my way,
for all my fellow *chingonas*
who don't like to follow the rules
but want to reap the benefits of
a happy and healthy lifestyle.

Let's do this!

# Glossary

**boss bee:** built on self-success (boss) babe embracing evolution (bee)

**cabrones:** the jackasses in our lives who we have to kick to the curb

**chula:** a beautiful, sexy, amazing woman

**lonja:** love handles, fat roll, muffin top

**nalgas:** your behind, butt cheeks, booty

**and . . .**

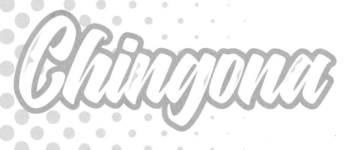

**a badass woman who lives life
on her own terms**

# Introduction

consider myself a *chingona*, and if you've picked up this book, I'm pretty sure you are a *chingona* too. Why? Because, like me, you bend the rules, you create your own path to follow your dreams, and you are ready to kick some *nalgas* and get shit done. I'm also guessing that if you are flipping through this book, you too have placed your health and body at the bottom of your priority list. It's easy to put ourselves last when we are juggling so many things in our lives, but that stops now. A crucial part of our badass journey in this world must include taking charge of our health, and that's what I hope we can do together with *Chi-Keto,* which is what I call my brand of keto, for short.

Let me guess: easier said than done, right? Yeah, I get it, and I'm with you. I know what it's like to grow up surrounded by family members who show their love through food and threaten you with the death of starving children when you don't want to finish the ginormous portions endearingly served on your plate. And what about the guilt trip that punctures our hearts when our *abuelitas* look at us with sad eyes because we are rejecting a second helping of our favorite dish, the one they spent the entire day making just for us? *¡Ay, Dios mío!* What do we do? We eat, that's what we do. We eat every last crumb on our plate. We learn to associate food with love and comfort, and when we're little and nicknamed *gordita* (otherwise known as "chubby" in Spanish), we learn to accept it as a term of endearment. Until we hit our teens and it all starts messing with our heads. If we're too thin, our family sets out to fatten us up to look "healthier," and if we're packing on the pounds, they warn us that we'll never find a man while looking like that, but they still feed us big-time, completely contradicting their ominous warnings. And so the dieting and yo-yoing begin.

Since I can remember, I have struggled with my weight. One time, I moved in with my *abuelita* for two months and gained a ridiculous amount of weight because I couldn't say no to her food—I would never disrespect my *abuelita* like that. It stopped one day, when my mom grabbed me by my newly minted love handles and said, "I think it's time for you to come home." But we struggled at home too. I grew up watching my mom and aunt try out different diets while my *abuelito* continuously told them what to eat and what to avoid. He was old school and super fit, and I know he thought he was giving out helpful advice when he'd say to my *tía*, "*Si estás gorda, no te va a querer un hombre.*" (If you're chubby, a man won't love you). I'm sure some, if not all, of you have heard a version of that line about not being able to get a man if you're packing on the pounds, either at home or at a family gathering. It's a classic in the Latino community, but it's far from helpful, am I right? All it really does is add to our already existing self-doubt.

As I came into my teen years, I not only got my mama's amazing genes (with curves for miles that I would eventually learn to love) but also some of her insecurities. That's when diets became a part of my life. And when I say I've done a lot of dieting, I mean, I've done it all, everything from the cabbage soup diet and juicing to no-carb and low-fat crazes. You name it, I've tried it. The first time I went on the Zone diet, it was with my mom's advice so that I could fit into my prom dress. And I went for it. I stuck to it for a month, lost the weight, felt like a queen in my dress, and when all the fun was over, I went back to my old eating habits and regained all the weight plus a few extra pounds. A moment of silence for the favorite jeans my thighs ripped. And, of course, the question that came from family members immediately after that . . . *¿y la dieta?* (and the diet?) And that's the cycle that continued with every diet since. I would do great at sticking to the plan, but after a while I'd start eyeing all the goodies my colleagues were having at business lunches or the tortillas, beans, and rice served at family gatherings, while I was stuck with a boring, flavorless piece of chicken, and it just got to me. Those bland, restrictive diets never fit my lifestyle. So I'd revert to my old eating habits and, after having sacrificed a month or two and seen the weight suddenly drop, I'd helplessly watch the scale go up, up, up, and away all over again.

Years of these ups and downs and the struggle with my weight began to take an emotional toll, especially when having to face it all in the limelight. From being bullied by the media to being trolled on social media, everywhere I turned there was always someone saying my booty was too big, my legs too thick, my face too round. The insecurities were already there, but I had been dealing with them in private; that is, until the media decided to shine a spotlight on all my physical flaws. And it hurt. Instead of learning how to embrace my curves and my body, I turned to hiding and covering them up. Definitely not a *chingona*'s mind-set, but hey, I'm human too. I felt like nothing would ever work for me, and I'd just shrug it off and think, *Let me just eat whatever I want and be happy.*

Sure, food calmed my anxiety and comforted me, but what I was eating wasn't really making me feel good . . . and I wasn't happy. I would wake up feeling tired, eat, and then all hell would break loose in my tummy. As I watched it bloat up like a balloon, I kept thinking, *Why is this happening?* I thought I was eating healthy food—frijoles, lentils, brown rice, egg whites—so why was my body not responding to these choices? And don't get me started on my clothes!

One of the biggest frustrations as a diehard fashion lover was not being able to fit into my favorite outfits. You know, one day we're strutting our stuff in our favorite jeans and the next day the damn zipper won't go up. I know you've been there, the jumping up and down, the lying on the bed, all the techniques to make those babies fit, until nothing works. And then denial hits. I'd tell myself, "Oh my god, this pair must have shrunk in the washing machine!" and with that, I'd retire them to the corner of my closet together with the rest of the clothes that no longer fit comfortably. The truth was I was making poor choices and eating too much. Denial is a prick! That's when my ride-or-die workout pants became my go-to outfit. Every morning I'd stand in my closet, glance over the jeans that choked me at the waist, and walk straight over to those unconditional workout pants. You know what I'm talking about, the ones that stretch with you so you don't really notice you are packing on the weight until it's too late. Girl, I started living in my workout pants; I'd use them every single day, and then go shopping for more, because you know I still wanted to look cute.

As if that weren't enough, I felt like I was dragging myself through each day, making a huge effort just to make it to nighttime to crawl back into bed. My schedule hardly ever lets up, so imagine having to jump from meeting to photo shoot to concert while constantly feeling hazy and drained. Yet just the thought of going on another diet was exhausting. Until it finally hit me: I can't live in these workout pants anymore. I can't limit myself like this. It's not making me happy. I like jeans, I want to change up my wardrobe, I want to feel comfortable wearing sleeveless shirts, I want to feel good inside and out. I knew it was time for a real change, one that I could turn into my lifestyle, and that's when I met my trainer and soon-to-be good friend, Sarah Koudouzian.

We instantly hit it off because she's a crazy *chingona* just like me. I loved the way she trained me, but if I had learned anything in my yo-yo years, it was that no amount of exercise would help if I didn't have a healthy diet as my foundation. So I turned to her, as

I'd done in the past with other trainers, and asked, "What should I eat?" And that's when I first heard the word *keto*. Keto is a high-fat, very low-carb diet that basically limits the amount of sugar that goes into your body to almost nothing so that instead of sugar, you use fat as an energy source. Sarah enthusiastically described that she'd been on a keto-inspired diet for the past year and a half and was in the best shape of her life. Coming from a trainer who didn't believe in counting calories or restrictive diets, and who was supportive of having mint chocolate chip ice cream once a week, I was definitely ready to give this keto thing a shot. I'm always willing to try new things, so the idea of trying keto didn't scare me.

There was a learning curve at first, so I texted Sarah a lot to make sure I was eating the right foods and making the right choices at home and on the road. "What do you mean I can have cheese?!" I said to her when she further explained keto to me. My mouth started watering. Not only could I have cheese, I could have butter and sour cream and . . . bacon! "What the heck? You're lying. This is a joke, right?" I couldn't believe my ears. I knew I had to do something to take control of my health again, but I never expected that would include cheese and bacon! Sarah then explained that all food was okay—the key was focusing on healthy sources of fat, which means olive oil, nuts, grass-fed and organic meat, chicken, and dairy, as well as wild-caught seafood. I was so excited. I couldn't believe I suddenly could have all these foods I had been told my whole life I would have to stay away from if I wanted to lose weight and keep the pounds off. For the first time ever I was able to picture actually maintaining a healthy lifestyle, and that's all I needed to jump right in.

Listen, after all my previous struggles with dieting, I accepted that I needed to find something that was going to work for me not just in the short term, but in the long term as well. I am going to have to watch what I eat for the rest of my life, and in order to do that, my meal plan has to be realistic and satisfy my taste buds. This is the first time I have really stuck to a "diet" and felt fulfilled. Scratch that, I don't even want to call it a diet because that word is filled with memories of restrictions, and diets in my mind have always been temporary rather than a path to a lifelong change. This is more like an all-day partay in your mouth.

Now let's be real: no matter how many delicious meals I had, of course I missed the carbs at first, but when I realized that I no longer had to eat bland egg whites and could instead have some of my favorite foods made with real Latin flavors *and* see weight-loss results, I mean, what more can a woman ask for?

Sarah patiently guided me through those first few weeks, recommending food choices, while also kicking my booty with exercises that had my muscles burning in beautiful agony. No pain, no gain, right? Despite feeling sore AF and experiencing some serious carb-withdrawal symptoms, by the end of that first week, I began to notice slight changes in my body and in how I was feeling. This alone already made my decision worth it.

Meanwhile, as I took off on my own personal keto journey and began sharing my experience with my followers, I also started noticing it was becoming super trendy on social media. However, some people who were following keto to the letter, counting every macro (short for macronutrient, the types of food we can't live without) and peeing on a stick to make sure they were in ketosis, or fat-burning mode, were reminding me of the more restrictive diets I've been on in my life. Don't trip, I'll dive deeper into all of this in chapter 1, but needless to say, that was not for me, and Sarah knew it. So we took the keto basics and Chiqui-fied them to fit me and my lifestyle. I steered clear of food logs and pee sticks, and she gave me the ultimate gift: an indulgence day once a week to satisfy any cravings so I could have my cake and eat it too—but just on Sundays, ladies! This is what makes this method different.

Although keto was booming, as I continued to share my journey with my followers, I realized Latino-food lovers had not tapped into it yet, likely because of the fear of eating fat being embedded in our heads, and because rice, beans, and tortillas are staples in the Latino culture. Can you imagine eating chilaquiles without the tortilla chips? (Don't worry, there's a keto-friendly recipe for you on page 54.) People were freaking out on me, worrying that I was eating my way to a definite heart attack with all these "fats" that for so long we've been trained to believe are bad for us. Funnily enough, that couldn't have been further from the truth. My digestive issues improved with the help of the extra fiber I got from the keto-friendly vegetables (yeah, I eat my veggies!), and I was feeling more focused, clearheaded, and energetic than ever before. For so long I had been searching for a way of eating that was beyond all diets, and the day had finally arrived: I had met my food soul mate. And now all I want to do is share this amazing experience with any-one and everyone who crosses my path, because it's delicious and it makes me feel sooo good. That's how Chi-Keto was born.

There are stacks of different keto books out there, but none really cater to our Latin culture, to the flavors we've grown up with, to the meals that we consider comfort food, and to our beautiful, curvy figures . . . except *Chiquis Keto*. In this book, you will find the keto-inspired recipes that make my mouth water and remind me of home, without the unnecessary carbs coming from tortilla chips or rice dishes like *arroz rojo*. Many of the recipes preserve our Latin flavors, but as a proud Mexican American born and raised in Long Beach, California, I love American food too. That's why, here, you will find everything from Chicken Taquitos (page 137) to Chocolate Blueberry Pancakes (page 62), which you can enjoy all while remaining healthy and learning how to eat the keto way: grain free, with good quality fats, moderate protein, and up to about 50 grams of carbs a day. Exactly what boss bees like us need to remain satisfied and focused on our goals.

The other key element to getting into a Chi-Keto frame of mind is Sarah's workout program. Her exercises celebrate our curves by lifting our booties and strengthening our God-given figures. And, on that note, baby girl, remember, there's nothing like embracing your beautiful body . . . flaws and all. Call one of your favorite girls and make a commitment to hold each other accountable. It's not only more fun to exercise with someone else, it encourages you to stop making excuses and skipping workouts.

I'll never forget the time, early on in our training, when a paparazzo approached my house to snap a photo of me working out in my backyard, and Sarah, noticing the scene, quickly removed her hoops and walked over to the gate and had her leave. I knew then and there that this crazy *chingona* was the real deal, and our training sessions soon became a place for me to let off steam, unwind, and even laugh and cry. She helped me accept that being fit is not about conforming to a specific look or size; it is about creating a healthy lifestyle and feeling great all around. This program will help show you how to embrace what's already amazing about your body and build on it, so you can strut your stuff with the confidence you deserve.

To get you feeling yourself the Chi-Keto way, there's one final component: the 21-day plan. Did you know that it takes twenty-one days to break and create a habit? That's right, three weeks, as in less than a month. I know we've all given some *cabrones* in our lives more days than that. So how about turning it around and devoting that precious time to ourselves and our health instead? All you have to do is commit to twenty-one days to form new, healthy habits and kick-start your very own Chi-Keto lifestyle. By the end of my 21-day plan, instead of being addicted to food, I was addicted to feeling good—the greatest inspiration to keep pushing forward. So get ready, queens! The next twenty-one days will be a mouthwatering adventure and an eye-opening reminder of how focused, driven, and energetic you can feel when you fuel your body with healthy food and work that booty to the rhythm of a great workout. You'll be seeing results in no time!

And I'll be with you, in these pages, every step of the way. I'm all about empowering women—we are so much stronger together, supporting one another, so let's make this another example of all we can accomplish hand in hand. Post your progress on Instagram, Twitter, or Facebook; hashtag it #ChiKETO; and I'll repost you. I got you, mama . . . and you got this!

*No more excuses, chulas: YOU are the priority.*

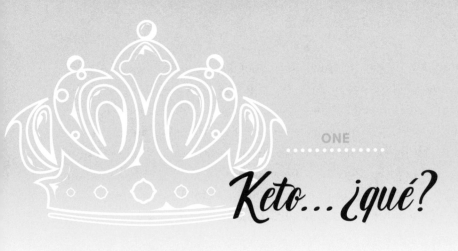

# ONE

# Keto... ¿qué?

Before we get on the Chi-Keto train to feeling fierce, it's important for you to understand the keto basics. So let's get down and dirrrty with the main concepts behind the ketogenic diet. Remember, I'm not a doctor or registered dietician, and this is not your standard restrictive keto book, so I'm not out to overwhelm you with scientific research and minute details explaining all the behind-the-scenes of a strict keto diet. You know how I roll, straight to the point. I just want to clear the information clutter and break down the keto basics for you so you can confidently take the next step to incorporating this way of eating into your life. However, if you want to learn more, I encourage you to talk to your doctor or a registered dietician and dive deeper into keto on your own terms.

## WHAT THE EFF IS KETO?

*Keto*, that word you see hashtagged everywhere in your feeds, is short for *ketogenic diet*, which is basically a very low-carb, high-fat, and moderate protein diet. The goal is to train your body to burn fat rather than carbohydrates because getting in that fat-burning zone will help you lose weight and improve your health.

In our carb-addicted world, our bodies have grown used to burning carbohydrates, which produce glucose to give us the energy we need to get through our days. This allows any excess fat in our body to cling to us like a stubborn *cabrón* who won't take no for an answer. Now if you lower your carb intake in a major way (as in less than 50 grams per day), your body will enter a metabolic state called *ketosis*. Being in ketosis (which usually takes a few days or longer to happen—results vary) means that without carbs for fuel, your body goes on the hunt for another energy source, and that's when the magic happens: it starts burning excess fat for energy, finally kicking that *bad boy* out of your temple. Ketosis helps turn fat in your liver into *ketones*, a type of acid, which are delivered to your bloodstream so that your body can use them as fuel instead of those pesky carbs that plague our existence.

Since carbs have been drastically reduced from the diet to reach this state of ketosis, and the body has turned into a fat-burning machine, it's important to up the amount of good, healthy fats in order to keep the body running smoothly. That's why the ketogenic diet not only calls for a very, very low amount of carbs but also for high amounts of fat and moderate protein. It's just teaching us a different and more efficient way to fuel our bodies.

## BREAKING DOWN MACROS: HIGH FAT, MODERATE PROTEIN, VERY LOW CARBS

Another word you see a lot in any keto-related post, article, or site is *macros*, which is basically a short and simple way of saying *macronutrients*. The three types of macronutrients—that is, the types of food required in large amounts because they are essential to our growth and health—are carbohydrates, lipids (aka fats), and protein. Different diets recommend different quantities of each of these macros to attain weight-loss results. The keto experts basically say that we should grab the current food pyramid and flip it, so that fats and proteins are at the base and now become the foundation of our diet. The standard ketogenic diet recommends 75 percent healthy fats, 20 percent protein, and 5 percent carbs. I know what you're thinking: it's hard to believe that we should actually be eating more fats, especially after years of having low-fat diet trends drilled into our minds. But it's time to throw that concept out the window and get with the times, ladies.

## YOUR NEW BFFs: *HEALTHY* FATS

That's right, fats are your new BFFs! You read correctly: healthy fats are actually . . . *good for you*! The problem is that most of us grew up during the low-fat craze that started in the 1970s when fat was suddenly linked to heart disease. Up until then, everyone had been enjoying meals that included full fats, but an abrupt shift in the food industry due to reports linking fats to heart issues turned our eating upside down and made *all* fats evil. The low-fat craze flooded our supermarkets, our TV commercials and shows, and our magazines, and we were trained to believe that this was the way to a healthier and longer life. What we didn't realize was that in order to keep the low-fat items flavorful, food manufacturers resorted to adding, among other fillers, sugar! So we replaced satiating full-fat food with crap that left us hungry and addicted to sweets. Not cute. Now I get why I always felt like I was craving everything in the world on previous diets!

But guess what? Most of the research done in the past twenty years has actually debunked the fats and heart disease link, so much so that even the American Heart Association (AHA) now embraces good fats, saying that they "lower rates of cardiovascular and all-cause mortality, lower bad cholesterol and triglyceride levels, provide essential fats your body needs but can't produce itself." I know this seems like a lot to take in, but the low-fat mentality is so ingrained in our society that it's important for us to become informed boss bees and realize what is up with what we're eating. There are two things I always preach: feed your soul and feed that mind, baby girl. Nothing is sexier than a woman who knows what she's talking about. If you want to read more on this, check out Dr. Mark Hyman's *Eat Fat, Get Thin*. He's done the extensive research from a medical professional's perspective and shares a wealth of information that explains why eating good fats is actually good for you.

So there you have it, but there's a catch . . . yeah, girl, I know, there's always a catch, but this one makes sense, so stay with me: not all fats are created equal. Medical professionals, scientists, researchers, and everyone and their mamas agree on one key point: trans fats are the enemy. So when we talk about upping your fat intake, this DOES NOT include any type of trans fats, such as the hydrogenated and partially hydrogenated oils found in vegetable shortening, margarine, fried fast food, commercially baked goods (yeah, I'm talking to you, donuts), potato chips, and so on. In a nutshell: if you limit your intake of processed foods that have a long-ass ingredient list on the nutrition label with words you can barely pronounce, you will be good to go.

Now let's get back to the good stuff, our new BFFs. The good and healthy fats that keto (and the AHA) recommend are the monounsaturated and polyunsaturated fats found in olive oil, avocados, salmon, and nuts and seeds. Keto also allows for saturated fats in small doses—I'm talking cheese, dairy, butter, and bacon, but keep them organic and grass fed, please. Keto, where have you been all my life? The key is to focus on the healthier fats to fill up your quota for the day—they fuel your body, aid vitamin absorption, help kick your sugar cravings, and keep you full. Use the saturated fats—a sprinkle of grass-fed cheese, a couple of uncured bacon strips, a dash of organic cream, or a sliver of grass-fed butter—to add flavor and keep you happy. If you're lactose intolerant, you can try low-sugar, low-carb dairy alternatives, such as soy cheese or low-sugar soy, almond, or coconut yogurt or cream. Here's a list that breaks all this down for you. Take a pic or bookmark it to keep it on hand as you learn your way around the Chi-Keto lifestyle.

## FATS: THE GOOD AND THE BAD

### Say YES to the Good Fats

Avocado (fruit and oil)
Cheese (full fat, organic)
Coconut (oil, milk, cream, butter, and MCT oil)
Eggs (organic, free range)
Fatty fish (like salmon)
Ghee and butter (grass fed)
Nuts and seeds (and their butters)
Olive oil
Olives

### Enjoy in Moderation

Cacao nibs (or dark chocolate)
Heavy whipping cream (organic)
Sour cream (full fat, organic)
Yogurt (full fat, Greek)

### Kick These Cabrones to the Curb

Canola oil
Corn oil
Grapeseed oil
Margarine
Peanut oil
Rapeseed oil
Safflower oil
Sunflower oil
Vegetable shortening

Protein is found all over our bodies—in our hair, skin, nails, muscles, bones, cartilage, tissues, and blood. It's a macro that our bodies don't actually store, so we need to have a regular daily intake to keep us healthy and strong, but that doesn't mean we have to binge on protein 24/7 to keep our bodies running smoothly.

Unlike the Atkins diet, which focuses on low carbs and high amounts of protein, keto calls for moderate portions of organic, grass-fed, or wild-caught protein in our meals to keep us healthy, full, and vibrant. The reason we don't want to overdo it with the protein actually has to do with how our bodies process it. If we eat more protein than what our body requires, it will grab that excess, turn it into glucose, and use it as fuel instead of fat, kicking us out of ketosis. That's why the key to protein intake in the keto diet is the word *moderate*. We'll get into portions in the next chapter, but for now, snap a photo or bookmark the following list so you know how to best pick and choose the protein that's right for you.

## PROTEIN

*Go For*

Eggs (organic, free range)
Fatty fish (wild caught)
Meat (organic, grass-fed beef, venison, pork, and lamb)
Poultry (organic, free-range chicken and turkey)
Shellfish (wild caught)

*Keep at a Minimum*

Processed meats (such as deli meat, salami, hot dogs, sausages, bacon). When you do indulge, make sure they are uncured, nitrate-free, and don't contain antibiotics.

*Beans may have protein but they are predominantly carb-loaded. If you love frijoles like I do, just set them aside and have a serving on your indulgence day. That's what that day is for!*

### JUST A LITTLE BIT—SOLO *UN PO-KETO*: CARBS

Ay, ay, ay, carbs, as much as I love you, you've gots to go! Well, not all of you, just grains, beans, lentils, starchy and root vegetables, and sugar. I know, in Latino cultures we're taught that our *comidas ricas* are also nutrient rich and good for us. Like the arroz and frijoles that we were told were filled with protein to make us grow big and strong. And no plate at home was complete without a side of *plátanos* and tortillas. But our *abuelitas* only told us half the story. What we didn't know is that all of these delicious staples are loaded with carbs, which turn into sugar in our bodies and spike up our insulin, creating mayhem all while we think we are eating food that is actually helping our health. You'll learn in the following chapter that on this plan you won't have to get rid of these classics forever; they simply become a treat that you can indulge in once a week.

However, not all carbs are bad. There's a list of low-carb foods that are actually not only okay but necessary to maintain a healthy balance while eating the keto way. That means you still have to fill up your plate with leafy greens or accompany your healthy fats and moderate protein with a side of cauliflower rice, broccoli, asparagus, or zucchini . . . trust me, girl, your body and booty will thank you!

Fruits are high in sugar, so they are considered a high-carb food, which keto advises to avoid. Yes, that means that *mangonada* (frozen mango magic) is definitely off-limits! But you can have a handful of berries (strawberries, blueberries, raspberries, etc.); just squeeze some lime juice and Tajín onto the mix and it'll be like you're not missing out.

On the keto diet, you are allowed anywhere from 25 to 50 net grams of carbohydrates. Listen, you already know I've been there and done that with the restrictive diets where you have to count every calorie or macro. And you'll learn in the following chapter that if you happen to overload my plate with spinach, so be it. But since we're talking keto basics in this chapter—and I know some of you just love your numbers, which is cool too—here's an easy formula to help you calculate net carbs when checking out a food label:

total carbohydrates – fiber – sugar alcohols = total net carbs

Most foods don't contain sugar alcohols, but rather only regular sugar. So in most cases, all you really have to do is subtract the fiber from the total carbohydrates and you'll get your magic number. This comes in handy as you adapt to the keto life. It's a real eye-opener when you start checking some of your favorite foods in the supermarket and realize how overloaded with carbs and sugar they are. Who would have thought that all those times I stopped at the local *frutero* stand to grab a "healthy" snack, I was actually loading my body up with more sugar than a can of soda?! To make it easier, check out the following list for the lowdown on Chi-Keto-friendly carbs.

## CARBS DOS AND DON'TS

*Eat Yo' Veggies*
Artichoke
Arugula
Asparagus
Bell peppers
Broccoli
Brussels sprouts
Cabbage
Cauliflower
Celery
Cucumbers
Eggplant
Green beans
Jalapeños
Kale
Lettuce (all types)
Mushrooms
Onions

Radishes
Spinach
Tomatoes (considered veggies from a chef's perspective)
Zucchini

### *Hello, Chi-Keto-Friendly Fruit*

Blackberries
Blueberries
Lemons
Limes
Raspberries
Strawberries

### *Sweeten It Up, Don't Sugarcoat It*

Monk fruit
Stevia
Sugar alcohols (sorbitol, mannitol, and xylitol)

### *Say NO to . . .*

Artificial sweeteners (Splenda, Equal, Sweet'N Low)
Bananas
Barley
Beans
Bread
Buckwheat
Cereal
Corn
High-fructose corn syrup
Honey
Oats
Quinoa
Pasta
Rice
Rye
Spelt
Sugar (white, brown, turbinado, coconut sugar, all of it!)
Starchy vegetables (potatoes, sweet potatoes, yams, plantains, and yuca)
Wheat

Alright, ladies, we've come a long way. Now that you know your macros and you've got your convenient lists of eat this and not that foods, it's time to take it a step further. As you now know, the standard keto diet is high in good fats (75 percent), moderate in protein (20 percent), and very low in carbs (5 percent). Sarah and I grabbed this macro breakdown and all the keto basics you've just read up on and Chiqui-fied them to keep it real and turn it into a way of eating that is easy to follow and maintain in the long run. What does this mean?

1. No more obsessing over counting macros à la strict keto.
2. Yes, yes, yes to learning how to make better choices so you know how to fill your plate with mouthwatering AND healthy food.
3. Hells yes to sweat sessions that get your body feeling good.
4. And the ultimate treat: one indulgence day a week to satisfy your cravings.

Flip the page to discover the Chi-Keto lifestyle and join me on this path to feeling effing fantastic inside and out!

*Glow on the inside, so you can shine on the outside.*

# TWO

# Keto My Way: I Don't Break the Rules, I Bend Them

I f you know me at all, one thing is for sure: I'm a *chingona* who doesn't break the rules, but I sure do bend them. I need to do things my way to get the results I want. And with keto this was no different. Peeing on sticks every day to obsess over my state of ketosis—been there, done that. Macro-counting, net carb–tracking, and food-logging—who has time for that? Not me, and I know you boss bees don't either.

Restrictive diets have never worked for me, and keto can feel very limiting and intimidating if you follow it religiously. I'm constantly on the move, on the road, hopping from a video shoot, to a business meeting, to a red-carpet event, to a photo shoot, to a concert. You name it, as the queen of multitasking, I'm doing it. Can you imagine me stopping in the middle of all that to pee on a stick or write down what I ate? It's just not going to happen. The minute I have to start counting crap and logging numbers is the minute I become disinterested and move on; it just doesn't fit my personality and my boss-bee life. Sarah helped me take the basics of keto and adapt the concept without obsessing over the numbers to better suit my lifestyle. I learned to connect with my body and with how I was *feeling*. Yes, as you progress in this journey, you will look great, but you will *feel* even better. From my many years of dieting, I can tell you one constant truth: if you work with a diet, the diet will work for you. But I was missing a crucial step: learning how to make it part of my life. As soon as I adjusted to my Chi-Keto lifestyle, my energy soared—I felt like I could fly. And that's what brought this all home for me.

You already know the keto basics, so how do we apply them in Chi-Keto? It's all about making it second nature, a way of life rather than a temporary fix. First step: finally saying buzz off to the numbers that plague our lives.

## NUMBERS BE GONE!

Why do we get discouraged and depressed when we try to improve our eating habits to lose some weight? Numbers, baby. We are so tied to the measurements and the numbers on the scale that we are letting those *números* define us. And when those numbers don't budge or don't reflect our sometimes unrealistic expectations—you know, like trying to fit back into your favorite dress after only a couple of days of consistent healthy eating—we throw our hands in the air and say, "*Ni modo*, this doesn't work!" and we give up. That stops now!

The only measurements you'll be taking on this 21-day plan are going to come from within. All I want you to do is concentrate on how you *feel*. I want you to learn how to eat without obsessing over counting calories or macros, and I want you to rejoice in the stunning energy levels and clarity of mind you will be experiencing rather than focusing on the number on a scale that isn't accurately reflecting your new way of life. Let me make myself extra clear: how you look is an extra perk that comes with this plan, but what I really want is for you to connect to how the Chi-Keto lifestyle makes . . . you . . . FEEL!

### How to Know What to Eat

All I need you to remember for Chi-Keto is that your plate should be 75 percent good fats, 20 percent protein, and 5 percent carbs. Sounds complicated, but it's sooo much simpler than you think, so stay with me, boss bee!

The goal here is for you to be able to easily calculate the portions on your plate so you keep a Chi-Keto balance without having to pull out the measuring cups and scales every time you want to eat. If you can easily identify the percentages on your plate, you won't need to track every single meal, and it will make eating out a no-brainer.

- **Protein:** All you have to do is use the palm of your hand to calculate the right protein portion on your plate. That's it. Regardless of whether it's a steak, a chicken breast, shrimp, salmon, or tofu, what goes on your plate should stick to the size of your palm.
- **Carbs:** Once you have the palm-size portion of protein on your plate, grab yo' greens and toss them liberally onto your plate. There are two places you should

always have greens: on your plate and in your pocket! Then add some low-carb veggies. Even a handful of berries as a snack is absolutely fine. You need veggies and fruit to maintain your overall good health, so don't shy away from these important staples on your plate.

- **Fats:** Okay, 75 percent sounds like a freakin' lot, I hear ya. But it's not, girl. Since we're now working with full-fat ingredients, you actually don't need that much to hit your recommended percentage.

Don't worry, each recipe in this book will teach you what a balanced plate of healthy keto-friendly food should look like, but just to give you an idea . . . picture your plate with your protein and all those yummy greens and/or low-carb veggies. Now drizzle some olive oil on the greens, add half an avocado, and sprinkle the dish with some seeds; or dress up the greens with some shredded cheese and a dollop of salsa and sour cream; or choose the holy grail of fatty protein, salmon, and accompany it with a low-carb veggie like asparagus and call it a day. Easy, right?

The key takeaway here is to forget about calculating macros and instead focus on filling your plate with high-quality, nutritious, and flavorful foods. Use the lists of good foods on pages 4, 5, 7, and 8, follow the weekly meal plans in chapter 3, and make the recipes in chapter 4—sticking to the suggested servings, of course. What's more, the food won't only look and taste great, you will actually be much fuller.

One of the main Chi-Keto goals is for you to become aware of what's on your plate and what you are feeding your body so you can keep yourself healthy. The emphasis is always on grass-fed dairy and organic meats and vegetables because food is fuel. The better the quality of fuel you put into your body, the better your body will respond in your day-to-day life. And, like a car, if you pump in too much fuel you'll drown the motor, so stick to the serving suggestions.

*The good fats and protein will help you feel full, and so will loading up on water. But don't shy away from the recommended snacks (see page 147) if you're hungry. Need a quick fix to hold you over till your next meal? Snack on a handful of pecans, walnuts, or almonds and you will be good to go. As a chingona, you may need to be reminded to starve your ego, but never starve yourself!*

### The Ultimate Backstabber: Your Scale!

First thing Sarah said to me before I started my keto journey was, "Get rid of your scale." She made it clear from the start: I had to forget about the numbers. "If you only focus on the number on the scale, all your attention will be on whether it is going up or down," she explained, emphasizing that my focus had to instead be on whether I was getting stronger, tighter, healthier. Yes, it may feel great when that damn number goes down, but when you've been doing everything right and that flashing number refuses to budge or suddenly shoots up, it feels like absolute crap and can even play a significant role in discouraging you from following your healthy eating plan. Truth time: I didn't get rid of my scale. I kept hopping on it like an addict, excited to see the number drop, until it stopped, and then it went up! My heart sank. I hadn't said anything to Sarah because I knew she'd give me shit for doing this, but I finally set my pride aside and texted her that I had gained two pounds. "How does that make you feel?" wrote Sarah. "So frustrated," I replied. "Now do you understand why I didn't want you to go on that backstabbing scale?"

When eating healthily and exercising à la Chi-Keto, we may be losing fat but we will also be gaining muscle and toning our bodies. This is actually something we should celebrate without the *pinche* scale getting in our way. Numbers can be deceiving and discouraging, especially for us women, since our weight fluctuates every single freakin' day. You know what I'm talking about. One day can make a two-to-three-pound difference on the scale, but the scale doesn't talk it out with you and explain that your hormones may be fluctuating or that you're bloating because of PMS (did you know women can gain up to five pounds during the days before their period?!). So we may be doing great with our eating and workout plan, but if that scale happens to reflect a different story, we feel that none of the effort and satisfaction we relished throughout the week was worth it. Think of the scale like that guy your mama told you not to date but you still decided to go out with only to find out later that he really was a lying douche. Take it from me, STAY AWAY from the scale—it will only frustrate and disappoint you in the end.

If you really want to measure your progress, check in with yourself on how you are feeling. Is your energy up? How are your clothes fitting? Are the exercises starting to get easier? Well, guess what? They're not getting easier, you are getting stronger! Something the scale won't ever tell you. Instead of letting numbers define you, put on a pair of pants that are a little too snug on you and snap a selfie, then use that same pair of pants in three weeks to snap another selfie so you can actually *see* how far you've come. We all know how much I love a good selfie, but nothing compares to seeing my progress shots, which show me how far I have come from just a few weeks ago.

After jump-starting my own Chi-Keto journey, I began to notice my facial features were more defined, my cheeks and tummy were less bloated, and my body was becoming stronger, and those small differences were so effing inspiring. By not using a scale, I learned how to focus on how I was feeling. I can't believe I used to be so attached to that number on the scale, which I now know took away from experiencing something amazing: the discovery of my own strength. I look back and think, *Damn, girl, all those times you gave up and look at you now!* I felt a difference in how my pants fit, then I dropped a dress size, and a while later another, and it suddenly hit me: I had finally flipped the switch and truly committed to taking control of my health. For someone who has been yo-yo dieting all my life, it took willpower and perseverance to finally realize that I am stronger than my excuses.

But hold up, this was far from an overnight miracle. It was a slow and steady process. Like the saying goes, "A candle that burns on both ends will not last the night." That's the epitome of what my other diets had been like, where I lost a lot of weight quickly and then packed it and more back on. The faster you lose weight, the quicker you will likely gain it again. "What comes easy won't last. What lasts won't come easy." I know, it sounds like one of your *abuelita*'s sayings, but it's so freakin' true! In this case, I am going slow, and I have lost weight, but the immediate difference is in how this lifestyle makes me feel, and that's what has encouraged me to continue the journey. The difference on the scale won't be as evident as the way your everyday clothes start to feel on your ever-improving body. Chi-Keto changed my perspective because it helped me take the spotlight away from the numbers and back on my overall health. I can't emphasize this enough: I feel healthier and more confident than ever before, and that's what I wish for you.

### Get It Right, Get It Tight

One time, I started following a new diet that actually said I had to steer clear of . . . exercise! The reasoning? Too much exercise could make you gain weight on the scale and that might discourage you to continue on the plan. Well, we already decided to toss that backstabbing scale aside, so forget this theory. In the Chi-Keto lifestyle, exercise is part of a healthy and balanced daily routine. Not only that, it's what helps you keep everything tight and looking good, *¿me entiendes?* (you with me?). I love feeling fit and tight, which is why I'm a huge advocate for working out (especially when we change our eating habits), and I want you to keep it tight too!

There's a workout plan for each of the three Chi-Keto weeks, and each individual exercise is detailed in chapter 5, with clear instructions on how to execute every move to feel like a queen. We'll get into all that later, but what I want you to remember now is the four Ds: a true Diva always remains Dedicated, Disciplined, and Driven! So make sure you keep your goals in sight and get at least thirty to forty-five minutes of cardio a day. And once you're done, congratulate yourself! I used to be so hard on myself, always obsessing over how I could've pushed harder and believing that what I did was never enough. But with this lifestyle, I stopped being so demanding. Now I actually congratulate myself even after a thirty-minute workout because I learned that getting through a set of exercises is a huge accomplishment.

Like every new habit, you have to give yourself time to incorporate it into your daily routine. Take your time with the workouts and go at your own pace, but promise me you'll move that booty at least a little each day and push yourself harder once you start to feel stronger. Is it tough? Hell yeah! But you got to get it right to get it tight. Is it worth it? Damn straight. You'll start feeling stronger, tighter, fitter, and more powerful than ever before. Will there be days you will want to give up? Um, yeah, and you know it. But those are the days you have to gather all that inner will, visualize all the good this is doing to your body and your life, and power through. If you tighten your shit up, when you start gradually losing weight, you'll discover muscles you didn't even know you had, and that alone will keep you motivated.

After a week's worth of hard work, healthy keto-inspired meals, and challenging sweat sessions, guess what Chi-Keto gives you that other keto diets don't? An indulgence day! Yes, you read right. Extreme restrictive diets just don't cut it for me. How do you sustain such hard and limiting rules for so long? Well, you don't. When I first started keto, I went all in, including the peeing on the stick. And even though Sarah had set up my indulgence day, I refused to take it, thinking strict keto was the way to go. Then, after two weeks, I caved and binged for a few days straight, until I finally began to snap out of it.

Constantly restricting ourselves makes us want to have whatever we've been prohibited from eating that much more. But I couldn't get out of my head the feeling that I was cheating on the indulgence day, and I feared that one day off would kick me out of ketosis and make me have to start from scratch the following morning. When I shared this with Sarah, she just looked at me and asked, "How many times are you going to fail on a diet before you realize this is a pattern for you?" Then she added something that stayed with me to this day: it's time to remove the phrase "cheat meal" from our vocabulary. The word *cheat* implies something bad, like we're undoing all the hard work we put in during the week by having this one meal. Enough is enough. That's why we call it an *indulgence* day, the key day that will help you turn this Chi-Keto plan into a lifestyle rather than a temporary fix. So let go of all that fear and simply enjoy . . . guilt free.

I chose Sunday as my indulgence day because it's usually my day off from work and when I spend more time with family and friends or simply squeeze in a little R&R at home. So on that day, I can visit my *abuelita* and eat her arroz con frijoles; or have lunch with my girlfriends and order a big ol' slice of cheesy, deep dish pepperoni pizza sprinkled with chili flakes to give it that extra kick; or share a banana split with my hubby; or simply indulge in some fettuccine Alfredo or whatever I was craving that week. Make sure to get some cardio in that day, like speed-walking, a jog, or putting on some booty-poppin' music to fit in a quick twerk session. But, pretty please, do not go overboard.

# Chingona Tip

## Treat Yo-self, but Don't Wreck Yo-self

Just because it's indulgence day doesn't mean you should binge on your cravings all day long. Pick one meal, one that you've been thinking about all week, one that makes your heart skip a beat, so that it's worth it, and make it your special indulgence, shamelessly savoring every bite.

Speaking of cravings, ever wonder why, after seeing a commercial with a happy bunch of people devouring a perfectly crispy-looking ten-piece chicken combo with a side of fries, you suddenly have the urge to order that for dinner? Because that's the ad's purpose: to toy with your mind and convince you that you can't end the day without having that food. And that's exactly what cravings do to you. They begin in your mind, something triggers a memory that leads to a specific craving, and then you just can't get it out of your head. But, remember, they're not something you need to survive, they're something your mind is telling you that you want. There's a big difference.

Listen, I'm not telling you to kick your craving completely to the curb. I'm just saying, acknowledge it but also recognize that you are strong enough to wait until your indulgence day to satisfy it. When your day finally arrives, simply replace one meal with the one that you've been craving—like chilaquiles with a michelada for lunch—or add a side of frijoles (can you tell that's what I miss the most!) to one of your dishes. Then eat your other Chi-Keto meals the rest of the day, which, by the way, are so good you might find you don't need much of anything else! If you're craving something sweet, stick to the meal plan and just add the dessert that you've had your eye on all week. If it's a cocktail you miss, go for the drink and stick to your keto-inspired meals the rest of the day. When a craving kicks in during the week, instead of feeling like you are prohibited from even thinking about that food ever again, you can now look forward to having it on your indulgence day. You feel me? Treat yourself, but don't wreck yourself, and hop right back on the Chi-Keto plan first thing Monday morning.

Breaking old habits is never easy, especially those that have been passed down from our *abuelas* to our *mamás* to us, like a hot tortilla and a side of beans. And creating new habits is equally hard, yet if it doesn't challenge you, it doesn't change you. But guess what? It only takes twenty-one days to create a new habit that can change your life for the better. I'm not saying it will all be fun and games. You *will* hit some roadblocks, because we're only human and shit happens. The first one to come a knockin' in week one will be the so-called keto flu. You'll also have to face temptations along the way and may have moments when you'll be close to caving. This is all okay. Don't beat yourself up and don't give it all up. Here are some ways to help you acknowledge these rocks and boulders in your path and bitch-slap them to the curb.

### The Keto Flu

During the first week eating à la Chi-Keto, it is likely you will experience symptoms that have been identified as the keto flu. When switching from a carb-loaded life to a keto-inspired eating plan, your body will be shifting from burning carbs for fuel to burning fat. That's wonderful, but while it is adjusting to your new way of eating, you will likely feel a little worse for wear before you feel better. When beginning any type of keto diet, it is normal to feel some, if not all, of the following symptoms:

- constipation or diarrhea
- fatigue
- headache
- insomnia
- irritability
- muscle cramps
- nausea
- upset stomach

It's normal because your body is in shock, trying to figure out where to find fuel now that you've eliminated carbs as its main resource. I'll be honest, that crap is not fun. That first week is a little tough. I remember feeling extra tired and having headaches. You may also get a little constipated or feel cramping or crave sugar as your body adjusts to not having sugar course through your veins anymore. Chin up and stick it out—it will only last a few days. I know you can do it. You just have to jump over this roadblock and keep going. In the meantime, here's what you can do to ease some of these keto flu symptoms:

- ***Stay hydrated, never thirsty.*** By cutting out most of the water-retaining carbs from your meals, you will be losing a lot more water as you adapt to this new way of eating. So up your water-drinking game with at least ten cups a day. To be more exact, calculate 75 percent of your body weight and that's the exact number of ounces you should drink per day.
- ***Replenish electrolytes.*** Electrolytes help keep you balanced, stave off muscle cramps, and ease keto flu symptoms. If you're not a hydrating queen, then you should up your intake of electrolytes during your first week on Chi-Keto until your body is able to adapt to this new way of fueling itself. Look for sugar-free (sweetened only with keto-friendly sugar replacements like stevia) and carb-free electrolyte supplements that contain the six essential electrolytes and minerals: magnesium, potassium, sodium, chloride, calcium, and phosphorus.
- ***Get your beauty sleep.*** Insomnia and irritability are common symptoms of the keto flu. So make sure to pull out all the stops to help your mind and body relax and get some rest. Cut down on caffeine, take a warm bath before going to bed, put down your cell phone, meditate, and go easy on yourself. You may have a night or two of restless sleep, but you will return to your normal sleeping patterns in a few days, so if all else fails, be patient.

Keto flu may be the first roadblock you encounter on Chi-Keto. I'll be honest: it's uncomfortable, and when you're experiencing it, all you want is for it to be over. Not everyone gets it, but if you do, hydrate with electrolytes, get rest, and go easy on yourself until it passes, because "this too shall pass." To get your mind to help your body through this tough moment, think of other instances where you've experienced a hard time in your life and how you coped till you got to the other side. I've had to push through many moments of pain—like when my mom died—to get better and be better, and I know you can too. Be patient with yourself. It won't last forever. Soon enough, you'll begin to notice the sluggishness and headaches lifting and giving way to a clarity of mind and focus that will have you wondering why you haven't done this sooner.

## WHEN TEMPTATION CALLS . . . AND IT WILL CALL

Temptation is the devil. Picture this: I'm onstage for two hours singing my ass off while throwing in an occasional twerk, followed by an hour of meet and greets. By the time I'm done, it's three in the morning and my ass is starving. All that's still open are fast-food restaurants and diners. When we walk in and sit down, everyone around me starts ordering hash browns, pancakes, French fries, milkshakes, double bacon cheeseburgers, and I'm about ready to throw my Chi-Keto ways out the door and dig into a damn burger. At first, resisting this bait was extremely hard, but once I learned how to satisfy my cravings without giving it all up, I actually took pride in defying temptation. The next time we pulled up to a drive-through, your girl caught the whole team off guard by ordering a keto-style cheeseburger, replacing the buns with lettuce and calling it a night. Remember, let your willpower be stronger than that temptation that won't do you any good. Resist, persist, and rejoice! Here're a few ways to help satisfy your cravings and keep temptation at bay:

| *Temptation* | *Solution* |
| --- | --- |
| Rice | Cauliflower Rice (page 113) |
| Frijoles | Keto Refried Beans (page 154) |
| Tostadas | Mozzarella Tostadas (page 80) |
| Tortillas | Chi-Keto-Friendly Tortillas (page 54) |
| Burger buns | Portobello mushrooms (page 85) |
| Pasta | Zoodles (spiralized zucchini) (page 122) |
| Elote | Cauliflower Elote (page 149) |
| Arroz con leche | Chia Seed Arroz con Leche (page 156) |
| Milk | Heavy whipping cream |

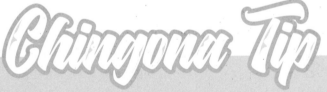

## Chingona Tip

### Don't Trade What You Want Most for What You Want Now

Chi-Keto offers plenty of alternatives that will get you the texture and flavor you are dying for without the extra carbs and sugar, so you can take control of your temptations and enjoy your craving on your indulgence day. Once you get used to eating this way, you'll notice your cravings subside too. So stay with it, honey.

I've been following my Chi-Keto lifestyle for more than a year now, and as much as I love it, I honestly still struggle when I go to my *abuelita*'s house. How can I say no to her frijoles charros? Do you know how damn hard it is to resist those creamy beans cooked in savory bacon with bomb-ass chorizo? It's not just that I don't want to hurt her feelings, it's also that I adore her food and it's part of the way we share our time together; that's why it's my ultimate temptation. Before I made this my lifestyle, I'd accept a heaping plate of food (or two, or three) from my *abuelita* and chow down until every last bite was gone. Now, with Chi-Keto, I've learned how to pick and choose what to eat when I visit her house and stick to *one* serving, leaving her famed frijoles charros for my indulgence day. I'm far from perfect, and sometimes I give in to temptation, especially when it involves my *abuelita*'s cooking. But I've learned not to beat myself up about it. We're only human, and we can't let one fall defeat us.

### Get Your Booty Back on Track

Losing our way can be discouraging—it's not our proudest moment, but it happens. It's when one temptation leads to a snowball effect: one slice of pizza here, two taquitos fritos there, a handful of chips in one hand, a cup of horchata in the other. Next thing you know, you're on your second week of that vicious cycle of self-sabotage with a sense of no return. It can happen when we get too busy and think we don't have time to cook up healthy meals. But it's not about having time, girl, it's about making time and putting in the effort. If you can't cook up one of the delicious recipes in this book, then take the Chi-Keto principles and apply them to whatever you order at a restaurant. Just cut the carbs, add the fat, and get back on track. Don't let a bump on the road detour you from your destination. Don't give up! Straighten your crown and get back to business.

During my first year on Chi-Keto, I had not one but two surgeries to deal with my ovarian cysts. In both instances, my medical team recommended that I follow what they believed to be a "balanced" diet to speed up my recovery. This included dairy (cool), meat (fine), and grains (hold up, we got a problem!). All I wanted was to heal, so I followed their advice and ate what they recommended for about a month. I did recover, but once I was ready to get back to my everyday life again, I didn't like how I was feeling. My energy was way down, my mind was foggy, and I was bloated again. I can't tell you how frustrated I felt. It was my biggest roadblock yet. My cheeks started getting puffy again (hey, I'll always be a little extra cheeky on the top and the bottom) and it crushed my spirit because I felt I had to start from square one. But as soon as I got the green light from my doctors, I hit the ground running (Sarah literally had me running for cardio) and faced that roadblock head-on like a boss bee! I felt I had lost an essential part of who I was and couldn't wait to come back to myself again.

After some struggles, I got my booty back on track and even twerked it out when I finally started rediscovering my long-lost energy and clarity of mind. That was all the motivation I needed to continue my Chi-Keto lifestyle. I'm at a point in my life where feeling good is my priority. I'm not getting any younger, and I want to continue to have the energy I need to get things done like a boss bee and enjoy a long, healthy, and prosperous life. I know it sounds crazy, and you won't truly grasp it all until you begin this journey yourself, but the minute you stop letting excessive amounts of carbs weigh you down, you feel so light and energized that there will be no looking back.

## LOVE YOURSELF EVERY STEP OF THE WAY

Everywhere we look, we are bombarded with images on social media of photoshopped and smoothed-out women who are pictured without a trace of cellulite or stretch marks, blemish-free skin, "perfectly" proportioned bodies, and not a *lonja* in sight. We are led to believe that this is what we are supposed to strive to look like. So we follow these guidelines, add a filter here, make a blemish disappear, and voilà, we are now the cookie-cutter example of what is considered beautiful in the media. Come on, we've all been guilty of falling into this trap. I know I have. The first step out of this mess is to recognize that this is actually a form of self-hate and self-sabotage. Ladies, we have enough haters doing this to us already. Why do we need to add fuel to the fire and do it to ourselves too?

Although I struggled with my weight at home, I honestly never really knew what an issue my body type would be in the public eye until I began working in television. That's when I was forced to confront the first wave of comments about my body: "You're too fat to be on TV. *¡Baja de peso!*" People insulted me and called me all kinds of names. The bullying was real, and I could sit here and pretend that I just ignored it all, but that's BS because I'm human, and words hurt, and I'm a hard shell with a soft heart. Truth: it got to me. I kept thinking, *Oh my gosh, is my body really that big of an issue?*

As the years passed, I developed negative voices in my mind that made me feel bad for not looking like what a public figure is "supposed" to look like. I was comparing myself to other people's *perception* and expectation of my appearance. And I started to believe them; I felt that in order to look better I actually needed to follow in someone else's footsteps. But aspiring to look like someone else only takes away from your own beauty and discredits who you are.

I didn't create the Chi-Keto lifestyle to conform to a certain number on a scale or look like someone else. I did it so I could learn to take care of my mind, body, and soul. But let's be real, sometimes those toxic inner voices can get the best of us. I still have days when I struggle with my body image and the insecure voices in my head. But I have finally learned to love and embrace my curves—and every dimple, scar, stretch mark, and wrinkle—no matter what the haters say. Your inner voices are always going to try and play you; self-realization is key to silencing those demons. Plus, a hater is always going to hate. In their eyes, we will always be too thin, too curvy, too tall, too short, or too much of something else. So we have to learn to love ourselves unconditionally, no matter what.

The Chi-Keto lifestyle has filled me with energy and positivity and has taught me to do away with unrealistic goals. I'm not aiming to be a size 0. My short-term goal was to lose a size or two to feel more comfortable in my own skin, but I don't want to get rid of my curves, only enhance them. They are part of who I am, and I am proud of that. I'm not eating to satisfy hunger. I'm eating to fuel my body so that I can fly through my day feeling great, energized, and able to accomplish my dreams. And I'm fueling my body so that I can accomplish my long-term goal of feeling fabulous and ultimately living a long and healthy life.

Set your own short- and long-term goals to celebrate every step of this Chi-Keto journey. Remember, *cada quien tiene lo suyo* (we are all unique), so trying to look like someone else does you no justice. We have to strive to improve our health and fitness because it's a form of self-respect. Your body is a permanent home for you to live in. What you put in it is what you'll get out of it. Nourish it and it will flourish.

*You gotta nourish to flourish.*

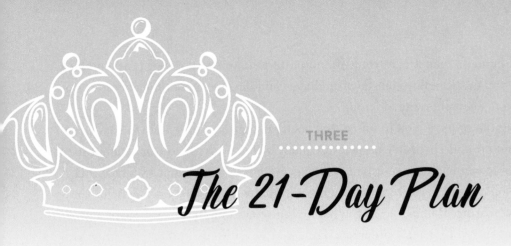

# THREE

# The 21-Day Plan

t's time for you to jump-start your Chi-Keto journey. Master the art of Chi-Keto by following the 21-day eating and exercise plan carefully mapped out for you in this chapter. Keep it simple. The goal is not to be perfect. The goal is to put in the effort every single day to help turn this new way of eating and working out into a healthy, lifelong habit. If you mess up and give in to a craving or skip a workout, don't let it turn into a "Oh, I'll just start again next week." Get it right for the rest of the day or pick up where you left off when you wake up the next morning. Change isn't easy, so please be honest and patient with yourself along the way.

This plan was designed to provide a clear guide of what to eat and how to work out efficiently. However, remember, Sarah and I are NOT medical professionals or registered dieticians. If you have *any* ongoing medical condition whatsoever, such as diabetes or a heart condition, please check with your doctor before starting this or any other diet.

We've taken the macro-counting and scale-obsessing out of the equation so that you can focus solely on creating the habits that will lead you to a healthy and vibrant life. With anything that we do, preparation is key. All you have to do is stock up on the necessary ingredients so you can prep ahead of time, follow the serving suggestions, and get in those workouts.

The recipes are interchangeable, meaning that if you prefer one breakfast over another, change it up and satisfy your taste buds. Same goes for the lunches and dinners. We've also provided snacks (see page 149) in case hunger strikes between meals. Some are sweet and some are savory to go with what you may need in that moment. Keep it to no more than one or two snacks per day, and only if you need them.

There's also a handy shopping list with everything you'll need to prepare each week's meals. Feel free to tailor the meals to your needs, schedule, and budget. The goal for this

Chi-Keto plan is not to complicate your life, but rather to help you create a new outlook that will allow you to still enjoy your favorite dishes and flavors without the excess carbs. I'm talking about a sensible way of eating.

By following the recipes, you'll notice that soon enough, you'll be able to easily recognize what should and shouldn't be on your plate without having to worry about food logs. Make sure to connect with your body and pay attention to it when it says basta. That signal saying you are full is easy to identify if you're listening, so stay in tune with yourself to avoid overeating. Remember, if you're craving something like there's no tomorrow, recognize it and save it for your indulgence day. And if you slip up and have a little extra something-something during the week, don't beat yourself up about it. It happens to all of us. Just find a way to balance it out, like adding extra cardio that day.

Each week's workouts are meant to be a challenge, but make sure you do them at your own pace. Push yourself, but listen to your body. Don't worry if you can't get through all the repetitions or all the sets the first time around. Simply do what feels right for you. With time and consistency, results will come. Just remember to be patient, consistent, and persistent. *Todo a su tiempo.*

And sometimes we like to celebrate accomplishments with a good ol' drink. Yeah, you read right. Did you expect a *tequilera* like me to adopt a lifestyle that didn't let me have my favorite tequila on the rocks? Whether you like it straight up, like me, or mixed, I got you covered in the Happy Hour section on pages 141 to 146. But hold up, *chingonas*, let's keep it real. If the goal is to lose weight, alcohol isn't the answer. So keep it to one or two drinks a week. That will keep you happy when chilling with your girls without undoing all your hard work. Bottoms up! *¡Salud!*

## Five Steps to Owning the Chi-Keto Lifestyle

1. Stick to real, whole foods, preferably grass-fed and organic poultry, dairy, and produce, and wild-caught seafood to up your nutrition game. Your body is a temple, mama. Invest in what you put into it.
2. Stay hydrated, not thirsty, queens! Drink lots of water throughout the day.
3. Get that booty moving and follow each workout at your own pace. Remember, it doesn't get easier, you just get <u>stronger</u>.
4. Never compare yourself to anyone because, <u>chula</u>, there's nobody out there like you. It's time to focus on your own personal goals.
5. You've got to nourish to flourish. We eat to fuel our body with good-quality nutrients, not to feed our emotions.

Once these three weeks are over, you will be a Chi-Keto queen serving up delicious keto-inspired meals without worrying about what to eat. It's time to boss-bee up and get this 21-day plan going!

*Less self-doubt. Más self-care.*

## THE CHI-KETO PANTRY

First up in prepping for your 21-day Chi-Keto plan is stocking up your pantry with all the goodies you need to spice up and season your new go-to dishes. If there's anything we Latinos know how to do really well is give food some *sabor*.

**Spices and Seasonings**

achiote

bay leaves

black peppercorns

chili powder

dried cilantro

dried oregano

dried rosemary

dried thyme

garlic powder

garlic salt

ground cinnamon

ground coriander

ground cumin

kosher salt

onion powder

paprika

red pepper flakes

sea salt

smoked paprika

taco seasoning

Tajín

vanilla extract

## Oils and Vinegars

apple cider vinegar

avocado oil

coconut butter

coconut oil

cooking spray

distilled white vinegar

olive oil

red wine vinegar

## Mustards and Sauces

Dijon mustard

grainy mustard

mayonnaise

pico de gallo

red enchilada sauce

salsa

## Canned and Jarred Chiles

chipotle in adobo

chopped green chiles

pickled jalapeños

## Miscellaneous

baking powder

baking soda

chia seeds

hemp seeds

sugar-free maple syrup

unsweetened coconut milk

unsweetened shredded coconut

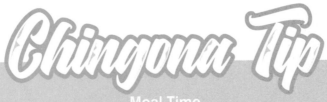

## Chingona Tip

### Meal Time

Spread your meals throughout the day, leaving two and a half to three hours between each one so you never feel like you're starving. Here's a sample meal schedule:

7:00 a.m.: Breakfast

10:00 a.m.: Snack

1:00 p.m.: Lunch

4:00 p.m.: Snack

6:30 p.m.: Dinner

Remember: Chi-Keto allows for one midmorning and one midafternoon snack, _but only if you need it_. Play close attention to what your body is telling you. Sometimes the body sends hunger signals when it's thirsty, so have a glass of water before reaching out for a snack and see how you feel. If you're still hungry, eat your snack (see recipes on pages 149 to 159), that's what they're there for. I get it, the struggle is real when you're trying to look like a snack while craving a snack.

# Rise and Slay

Congratulations for taking the first step to a healthier and upgraded version of you! I'm so proud you decided to join me on this Chi-Keto 21-day plan. As you probably know from your own life experiences, change is a challenge, and so is this first week entering Chi-Keto. You will be replacing your regular carb-loaded way of eating with food that will efficiently fuel your body, which is amazing, but not before going through the keto flu feels. Remember to drink LOTS of water to help flush out toxins and keep you full as you get used to eating the Chi-Keto way.

## Chingona Tip

If you're trying to satisfy that sweet tooth (especially if it's that time of the month), try one of the snacks on pages 149 to 159.

The Chia Seed Arroz con Leche (page 156) is my fave!

It's time to boss up! Always keep your priorities in check and your head up so that crown doesn't fall.

## CHI-KETO MENU—WEEK 1*

If you're hungry between meals, we've got your sweet and savory teeth covered with the snack recipes on pages 149 to 159. It is okay to have one or two snacks per day (one midmorning and/or one midafternoon) *if needed*, meaning if you need a little extra kick to keep you satisfied until your next meal. Just make sure to follow the recipe's recommended serving.

### Day 1
Breakfast: Huevos Rancheros (page 53)
Lunch: Aguachile (page 79)
Dinner: Chi-Keto Tacos (page 111)

### Day 2
Breakfast: Chorizo Breakfast Bowl (page 56)
Lunch: Chile Gordo (page 81)
Dinner: Fajitas a la Flor (page 113)

### Day 3
Breakfast: Aguacate Relleno (page 57)
Lunch: À la Chi-Taco Salad (page 82)
Dinner: Nacho-Bitch (page 115)

### Day 4
Breakfast: Chi-Muffins (page 58)
Lunch: Not Your Basic Chick (page 84)
Dinner: Shrimp Ceviche with Keto Tostada (page 116)

### Day 5
Breakfast: Fajita Frittata (page 59)
Lunch: Chi-Keto Burgers (page 85)
Dinner: Pollo a la Plancha (page 117)

* In a celebratory mood? Check out the Happy Hour section (pages 141 to 146). Just make sure you stick to the recipe's recommended serving and keep it to one or two drinks a week.

## Day 6

Breakfast: Chi-Keto Horchata Smoothie (page 60)
Lunch: Carnitas with Jalapeño Poppers (page 86)
Dinner: Roasted Salmon with Lime Cream Sauce and Asparagus (page 118)

## Day 7

Breakfast: Chilaquiles con Chicharrón and Avocado Crema (page 61)
Lunch: Steak Fajita Salad with Cilantro Lime Dressing (page 88)
Dinner: Fried Chicken with Mashed Garlic Cauliflower (page 120)

## SHOPPING LIST—WEEK 1

We made your life easier and created a shopping list of all the things you will need to prepare your meals each week. Because if you're prepared, you will succeed!

### Dairy

Colby Jack cheese
cream cheese
eggs
garlic ghee
ghee
grass-fed butter
grated Parmesan
half-and-half

heavy cream
Mexican crema
queso blanco
shredded cheddar cheese
shredded Cotija cheese
shredded mozzarella
sour cream

### Produce

arugula
asparagus
avocados
baby spinach
butter lettuce
cantaloupe wedges
cauliflower heads
cauliflower rice

chives
cilantro
cucumber
garlic
green bell peppers
jalapeños
lemons
limes

navel orange

parsley

poblano peppers

portobello mushrooms

radishes

raspberries

red bell peppers

red onions

Roma (plum) tomatoes

romaine lettuce

scallions

serrano peppers

strawberries

white onions

yellow bell peppers

yellow onions

## Seafood and Meat

bacon

boneless pork shoulder

boneless, skinless chicken breasts

chicken legs (drumsticks and thighs)

flank steak

ground chicken

ground turkey (85% lean)

ham

large shrimp (peeled and deveined)

sweet or hot Mexican chorizo

## Miscellaneous

blanched almonds

canned diced tomatoes

chicharrón

chicken broth

dark beer

egg white protein powder

extra-virgin coconut butter

sliced pickled jalapeños

unsweetened almond milk

unsweetened coconut milk

The distance between where you are and where you want to be is determined by how badly you want it. Is it easy? No. But it's so damn worth it!

**Workout/Twerkout Playlist**
"Booty"—Becky G featuring C. Tangana
"Booty"—Jennifer Lopez featuring Iggy Azalea
"She Bad"—Cardi B and YG
"Cristina"—Maffio featuring Nacho, J Quiles, and Shelow Shaq
"Good Form"—Nicki Minaj featuring Lil Wayne
"Dinero"—Jennifer Lopez featuring DJ Khaled and Cardi B
"Money"—Cardi B
"200 MPH"—Bad Bunny featuring Diplo
"0 to 100 / The Catch Up"—Drake
"Martes es muy lejos"—Chiquis

For more info on how to properly do each move, see chapter 5: The 12 Essential Exercises for a *Chingona*'s Body.

Workout 1
Glute Bridges 10 reps × 3 sets
Banded Bicep Curls 12 reps × 3 sets
Banded Squats 10 reps × 3 sets
Plank 20 seconds × 3 sets

Workout 2
Stagnant Lunges 12 reps × 3 sets
Push-Ups 10 reps × 3 sets
Back Rows 10 reps × 3 sets
Crunches 15 reps × 3 sets

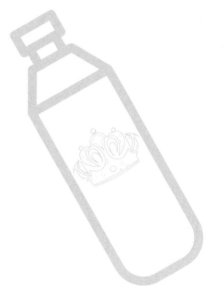

Mountain Climbers 15 seconds × 3 sets
Shoulder Presses 10 reps × 3 sets
Glute Kickbacks 12 reps × 3 sets
Tricep Kickbacks 10 reps × 3 sets

*Yass, queen, you made it!*
*Look at you completing week one like*
*the powerful woman that you are . . .*
*don't stop now!*

# The Best View Comes After the Hardest Climb

The hardest part of anything we do is to start. Week one may have been tough, but mama, you just proved that you're tougher. By week two, I began to look forward to my next meal and realized that this exercising and healthy eating thing wasn't so bad. I got the hang of what I should and shouldn't eat and you will too. You'll now start to feel more in control of the food and the workouts and even notice a shift in your energy.

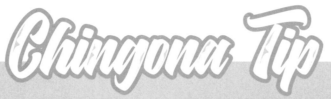

## Chingona Tip

*I know you may still be missing certain foods, like tortillas. Girl, I was too! There's nothing like homemade tortillas, but I got you with a bomb keto-friendly tortilla recipe (page 54) that you can enjoy with the Chicken Chipotle Casserole (page 94) lunch featured in day 11 this week!*

*Keep grinding because at the end you'll be thriving.*
*Repeat after me: I'm doing this for me.*

## CHI-KETO MENU—WEEK 2*

Remember, if you're hungry between meals we've got your sweet and savory teeth covered with the snack recipes on pages 149 to 159. It is okay to have one or two snacks per day (one midmorning and/or one midafternoon) *if needed.* Just make sure to follow each recipe's recommended serving.

### Day 8

Breakfast: Chocolate Blueberry Pancakes (page 62)
Lunch: Chicken Tortilla Soup (page 90)
Dinner: Creamy Chicken Tomato Noodles (page 122)

### Day 9

Breakfast: Blueberry Cheesecake Bar (page 63)
Lunch: Prosciutto Arugula Pizza (page 91)
Dinner: Chicken Sausage Vegetable Skillet (page 123)

### Day 10

Breakfast: Machaca con Huevos (page 64)
Lunch: Ground Turkey Stuffed Avocados (page 93)
Dinner: Chicken Enchilada Bowl (page 124)

### Day 11

Breakfast: Coconut Pancakes (page 65)
Lunch: Chicken Chipotle Casserole (page 94)
Dinner: Carne Asada with Chimichurri in Lettuce Wraps (page 125)

### Day 12

Breakfast: Ham and Cheese Omelet Stuffed in Bell Pepper (page 66)
Lunch: Pollo en Mole Verde with Hemp Seed Rice (page 95)
Dinner: Costillas de Puerco en Adobo con Ensalada de Nopales (page 127)

* In a celebratory mood? Check out the Happy Hour section (pages 141 to 146). Just make sure you stick to the recipe's recommended serving and keep it to no more than one or two drinks a week.

## Day 13

Breakfast: Bacon Avocado Bomb (page 67)
Lunch: Pechuga de Pollo en Salsa de Queso y Espinaca (page 97)
Dinner: Carne a la Tampiqueña with Roasted Zucchini (page 129)

## Day 14

Breakfast: Blueberry Chia Pudding (page 68)
Lunch: Chile Relleno with Ground Chicken (page 98)
Dinner: Filete de Pescado with Cucumber and Cheese Salad (page 131)

## SHOPPING LIST—WEEK 2

One of my favorite hobbies is shoe shopping. I never thought grocery shopping would make the cut, but cooking became therapeutic for me; I was finally in control of what I was putting in my body. It's so much easier to maintain your healthy way of eating if you shop for your ingredients ahead of time!

### Dairy

cream cheese
eggs
heavy cream
garlic ghee
grass-fed butter
grated Parmesan
Monterey Jack cheese

ranchero cheese
shredded cheddar cheese
shredded Cotija cheese
shredded Mexican cheese blend
shredded mozzarella cheese
  (low-moisture)
sour cream

### Produce

Anaheim chiles
arugula
avocados
basil
baby spinach
butter lettuce
cauliflower

cauliflower rice
celery stalks
chives
cilantro
cremini mushrooms
fresh blueberries
frozen blueberries

garlic
jalapeños
lemons
limes
nopales (cactus pads)
parsley
pasilla chiles
Persian (mini) cucumbers
portobello mushrooms
radishes

red bell peppers
red onion
Roma (plum) tomatoes
romaine lettuce
scallions
serrano peppers
tomatillos
white onions
zoodles (spiralized zucchini)
zucchini

## Seafood and Meat

baby back ribs
bacon
boneless, skinless chicken breasts
boneless, skinless chicken thighs
chicken legs (drumsticks and thighs)
dry beef (jerky)
flank steak

fresh chicken sausage links
ground chicken
ground turkey (85% lean)
ham
prosciutto (nitrate-free)
tilapia fillets
skirt steak

## Miscellaneous

ancho chiles
carb-free chocolate protein
chia seeds
chicken broth
cinnamon stick
coconut flour
dark chocolate (at least 70% and
   unsweetened)
dried basil
dried parsley

erythritol
guajillo chiles
hemp seeds
hulled pumpkin seeds
Italian seasoning
low-carb tortillas
Moon cheese
pine nuts
sliced almonds
sundried tomatoes in oil

During my second week working out with Sarah, I thought, *Oh my gosh, what am I doing?* She was literally a pain in my *nalgas*—every time I got up from the couch or toilet, I lovingly cursed her because I felt muscles I didn't even know I had. You don't know real struggle until trying to pull up your jeans after a leg and booty workout!

**Workout/Twerkout Playlist**
"La Hora Loca"—Jackie Cruz
"Con Altura"—Rosalía and J Balvin
"Get up 10"—Cardi B
"No Limit"—G-Eazy featuring Cardi B and A$AP Rocky
"ReBoTa"—Guaynaa
"Love Don't Cost a Thing"—Jennifer Lopez
"Megatron"—Nicki Minaj
"Ovarios"—Jenni Rivera
"Level Up"—Ciara
"Completamente"—Chiquis

For more info on how to properly do each move, see chapter 5: The 12 Essential Exercises for a *Chingona*'s Body.

## Workout 1

Banded Glute Bridges 15 reps × 3 sets
Dumbbell Bicep Curls 12 reps × 3 sets
Plank 30 seconds × 3 sets
Dumbbell Squats 12 reps × 3 sets

## Workout 2

Modified Push-Ups 12 reps × 3 sets
Alternating Lunges 10 reps × 3 sets
Crunches 20 reps × 3 sets
Single-Arm Back Rows 12 reps × 3 sets

## Workout 3
Mountain Climbers 25 seconds × 3 sets
Alternating Shoulder Presses 12 reps × 3 sets
Banded Glute Kickbacks 15 reps × 3 sets
Tricep Kickbacks 12 reps × 3 sets

*Believe in the woman you are becoming.*
*The only time you should look back is*
*to see how good your booty is lookin'!*

# Take a Moment to Appreciate How Far You've Come

By week three, we start to notice some changes in our bodies and our confidence. And with that we become more comfortable: "Oh, my clothes are starting to fit looser, so it's okay for me to have that piece of cake today." Then tomorrow comes and we say, "Well, since my clothes still feel loose, that means I lost some weight, so I deserve those French fries. Plus, I'm going to burn it all off later with my workout." Sound familiar? *¡No te dejes,* mama*!* Don't let this happen to you! Stay focused on your goals and finish this plan strong.

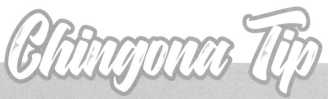

## Chingona Tip

Sometimes what's harder than starting something is finishing it. Think back and remind yourself of why you began this journey!

Motivation is what gets you started.
Habit is what keeps you going!

## CHI-KETO MENU—WEEK 3*

By week three, your need for snacks will likely be at a minimum. But if you're hungry between meals, we've got your sweet and savory teeth covered with the snack recipes on pages 149 to 159. Keep it to no more than one or two snacks per day (one midmorning and/or one midafternoon) *if needed* and follow each recipe's recommended serving.

### Day 15
Breakfast: Sausage Torta (page 69)
Lunch: Chicken Cheese Quesadilla (page 99)
Dinner: Camarones a la Diabla with Mexican Kale Salad (page 132)

### Day 16
Breakfast: Chi-Keto Pancakes (page 70)
Lunch: Spicy Mozzarella Chicken Burger Ranch Salad (page 100)
Dinner: Mexican Meatsa (page 134)

### Day 17
Breakfast: Portobello Egg Toast (page 71)
Lunch: Stuffed Zucchini Boats (page 102)
Dinner: Lemon Pepper Chicken Wings with Ranch Dressing (page 135)

### Day 18
Breakfast: Cheesy Turkey Egg Tacos (page 72)
Lunch: Tuna Bacon Salad (page 103)
Dinner: Coconut Chicken Tenders (page 136)

### Day 19
Breakfast: Crispy Cinnamon Almond Waffles (page 73)
Lunch: Steak Fajita Rolls (page 104)
Dinner: Chicken Taquitos (page 137)

* Feel like celebrating? Check out the Happy Hour section (pages 141 to 146). Just make sure you stick to the recipe's recommended serving and keep it to no more than one or two drinks a week.

**Day 20**

Breakfast: Pumpkin Spice Coffee Smoothie (page 74)
Lunch: Bacon Guacamole Chicken Bomb (page 105)
Dinner: Broiled Salmon with Arugula Salad (page 138)

**Day 21**

Breakfast: Chocolate Green Creamy Smoothie (page 75)
Lunch: Shrimp Stir-Fry (page 107)
Dinner: Chili for the Soul (page 139)

## SHOPPING LIST—WEEK 3

By now, your grocery store is your second home, and you know what you need to fill up your plates with Chi-Keto food, so tailor your shopping list to your liking and stock up on your favs and must-haves for Monday.

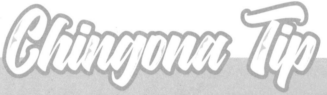

*Never go to the grocery store hungry. You'll end up in the panadería section loading up your cart with pastries and pan dulce.*

### Dairy

cream cheese
eggs
ghee
grass-fed butter
grated Parmesan cheese
Mexican cheese blend

Mexican crema
shredded cheddar cheese
shredded mozzarella cheese
  (low moisture)
sour cream
vanilla ghee

### Produce

avocados
baby arugula

baby bella mushrooms
baby kale

baby spinach
broccoli florets
carrots
celery
cilantro
dark leafy greens
dill
fresh rosemary
fresh thyme
garlic
green bell peppers
iceberg lettuce
jalapeños

lemons
limes
parsley
Persian (mini) cucumber
portobello mushrooms
red onions
Roma (plum) tomatoes
scallions
shallot
white onions
yellow bell peppers
yellow onions
zucchini

## Seafood and Meat

bacon
boneless, skinless chicken breasts
chicken tenders
cooked turkey breast
chicken wings
ground beef (85% lean)
ground chicken

ground turkey (85% lean)
large shrimp (peeled and deveined)
salmon fillets
sausage patties
sirloin steak
tuna packed in olive oil

## Miscellaneous

beef broth
cashew flour
dried chives
instant coffee
liquid aminos
loose chai tea
pitted black olives
raw unsweetened cacao powder

sesame seeds
superfine almond flour
sriracha
toasted sesame oil
turmeric
unsweetened coconut cream
unsweetened pumpkin puree
Worcestershire sauce

When I reached this week, I just remember thinking, *It hurts so good!* I could not only feel the difference, I started to see it. Mind's strong, body's strong, so we finish strong!

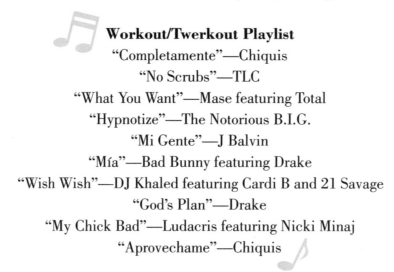

**Workout/Twerkout Playlist**
"Completamente"—Chiquis
"No Scrubs"—TLC
"What You Want"—Mase featuring Total
"Hypnotize"—The Notorious B.I.G.
"Mi Gente"—J Balvin
"Mía"—Bad Bunny featuring Drake
"Wish Wish"—DJ Khaled featuring Cardi B and 21 Savage
"God's Plan"—Drake
"My Chick Bad"—Ludacris featuring Nicki Minaj
"Aprovechame"—Chiquis

For more info on how to properly do each move, see chapter 5: The 12 Essential Exercises for a *Chingona*'s Body.

### Workout 1

Glute Bridges to Chest Presses 15 reps × 3 sets
Plank 45 seconds × 3 sets
Squats to Shoulder Presses 12 reps × 3 sets
Alternating Bicep Curls 15 reps × 3 sets

### Workout 2

Plank Rows 10 reps × 3 sets
Crunches 25 reps × 3 sets
Stagnant Lunges to Bicep Curls 10 reps × 3 sets
Push-Ups 8 reps × 3 sets

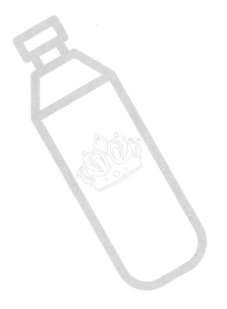

Mountain Climbers 30 seconds × 3 sets
Squats to Shoulder Presses 15 reps × 3 sets
Banded Glute Kickbacks 15 reps × 3 sets
Banded Tricep Kickbacks 15 reps × 3 sets

Congratulations, chula!
You may have struggled in
the beginning, but you didn't quit.
You're the true definition of a chingona!
Now take what you learned and keep going.
Use hashtag #ChiKETO so I can see your progress!

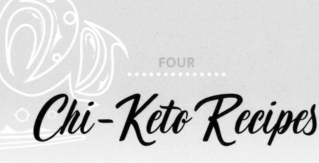

# FOUR

# Chi-Keto Recipes

Listen, I understand a *chingona* is always on her hustle game; you stay on the go balancing work, friends, and *la familia*. To save you some time and extra work, here are some tips to speed up your cooking process!

1. Go grocery shopping and prep your meals in advance for the week.
2. Stick to the suggested servings for each recipe to stay on track, and if you're hungry between meals, have a snack.
3. If a recipe calls for any of the following, you can purchase the premade version from the store:
   - Cauliflower tortillas
   - Cauliflower pizza crust (must be under 10 grams of carbs)
   - Store-bought salsa (no sugar added)
   - Store-bought pico de gallo (no sugar added)
   - Store-bought frozen or fresh prepackaged zoodles
   - Store-bought frozen or fresh prepackaged cauliflower rice
   - Ready-made rotisserie chicken

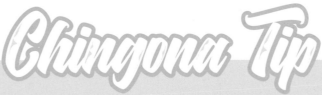

*If you fall offtrack for the day, don't beat yourself up. Setbacks are opportunities to learn from the fall and come back stronger. Let it go and get back on it for the next meal.*

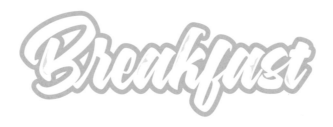

# Breakfast

*God morning, you beautiful soul! Nothing like a satisfying breakfast to fill you with energy so you can get off on the right track. I like to use my mornings to set the tone for the day and manifest what I want to accomplish, boss-bee style. If I have a hectic day ahead, I'll go for the Bacon Avocado Bomb (page 67) because it's quick and easy to eat in the car. When I have a few morning minutes to spare, I'll get down with the Huevos Rancheros (page 53) and savor every delicious bite—it's my comfort food and it feels like home. Remember, you can follow the weekly meal plans in chapter 3 or you can pick and choose whatever breakfast your schedule or mood desires.*

## Chingona Tip

No need to do without your morning coffee on Chi-Keto. Just keep it black, add a spoonful of MCT oil to up your health factor, and if you take it sweet, use a natural sweetener like stevia or monk fruit. If <u>café con leche</u> is your jam, feel free to add a splash of heavy whipping cream or nut milk or coconut milk, just make sure to avoid milk, which has more sugar, meaning more carbs.

# *Huevos Rancheros* (Eggs with Tomato Sauce)

This is one of my favorite recipes because it brings me back to when I was about twelve years old, living with my mom, who was pregnant with Jenicka, and stepdad, Juan, off Keene Street in Compton. Every Saturday we used to wake up and clean the house. Toward the end of our cleaning session, my mom would head over to the kitchen and start making her huevos rancheros, which was a dish my stepdad always craved back then. The music was playing in the background. I remember like it was yesterday the smell and sound of the tortillas frying in the pan and how excited I was to get that reward after cleaning. Until then, I had grown up with my crazy single mom doing everything in her power to survive, but during that time she had become a full-blown mother, pregnant with my sister and devoted to my stepdad. Sitting around the table devouring those eggs together was the first time I felt like we were actually a family.

SERVES 1
PREP TIME: 10 minutes
COOK TIME: 45 minutes

1 tablespoon garlic ghee
2 large eggs
2 Chi-Keto-Friendly Tortillas
  (page 54)
Tomato Sauce (page 55)
½ avocado, halved, pitted, peeled,
  and diced
2 tablespoons shredded Cotija cheese
Cilantro leaves, for garnish

1. In a small pan, heat the ghee over medium heat. Crack the eggs into the pan and cook until the whites are set.
2. Place the tortillas on a plate and top with the eggs, 3 to 4 tablespoons tomato sauce, the avocado, and cheese. Garnish with cilantro leaves.

## Chi-Keto-Friendly Tortillas

Keep this keto-friendly tortilla recipe handy. It's so good you can even share it with your *abuela*! So when a recipe calls for tortillas use this!

**MAKES 12 TORTILLAS**
**PREP TIME:** 10 minutes
**COOK TIME:** 15 minutes

4 ounces plain chicharrón (about 5 cups)
⅛ teaspoon baking soda
⅛ teaspoon kosher salt
3 cold large eggs (make sure they're cold!)
3 large egg whites
4 ounces cream cheese, softened
¾ cup plus 2 tablespoons cold water
3 tablespoons olive oil
Cooking spray

1. In a food processor, finely process the chicharrón with the baking soda and salt. Add the eggs, egg whites, cream cheese, ¾ cup water, and the oil and process until well combined.
2. Transfer to a bowl and let stand until the consistency of honey, about 5 minutes.
3. Spray a medium nonstick pan with cooking spray and heat over medium heat until hot.
4. Pour ¼ cup of the batter into the pan and use a spoon or offset spatula to spread it into a 6-inch circle (it should be thin). If the batter gets too thick, add one tablespoon of the remaining water at a time to thin it to the proper consistency. Cook until golden brown, about 30 seconds, then flip the tortilla over and cook until the underside is golden brown, about 30 seconds more. Repeat with the remaining batter, stacking the tortillas on a plate as they're finished. Pay close attention as they cook fast!

## Tomato Sauce

MAKES 1 CUP
PREP TIME: 10 minutes
COOK TIME: 30 minutes

3 Roma (plum) tomatoes
½ medium white onion, coarsely chopped
½ jalapeño, or more if desired (ribs and
 seeds removed for less heat, if desired)
1 clove garlic
Kosher salt to taste

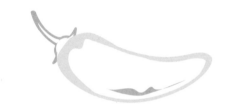

1. Preheat the oven to 400°F.
2. On a small rimmed sheet pan, roast the
 tomatoes until softened, about 20 minutes. When cool enough to handle, use
 your finger to peel them and discard the
 skin.
3. In a blender, puree the tomatoes, onion,
 jalapeño, and garlic until smooth; season with salt.
4. Transfer to a medium saucepan and
 cook over medium-low heat, stirring
 frequently, until sauce no longer tastes
 of raw onion, about 10 minutes.

# Chorizo Breakfast Bowl

Chorizo is a must-have staple in any Latino household—the spicier the better for me. This is a great savory combo of good fats, proteins, and low-carb veggies that will keep you satisfied and thriving throughout the morning.

**SERVES 2**
**PREP TIME:** 5 minutes
**COOK TIME:** 7 minutes

1 tablespoon ghee
3½ ounces fresh sweet or hot Mexican chorizo (1 link), casing removed
2 large eggs
¼ cup half-and-half or heavy cream
½ cup shredded cheddar cheese
1 small tomato, diced
½ small yellow onion, diced
½ avocado, pitted, peeled, and diced
1 to 2 tablespoons sour cream
2 tablespoons chopped cilantro

1. In a small skillet, heat the ghee over medium heat. Add the chorizo, crumble it with a fork, and cook, stirring occasionally until cooked through, about 3 minutes. Reduce the heat to medium-low. Divide half the chorizo between two bowls and set the remaining half aside.

2. In a small bowl, whisk the eggs with the half-and-half, add to the skillet, and cook, stirring constantly until the eggs are set but still soft, about 3 minutes.

3. Divide the eggs between the two bowls and top with the cheese, reserved chorizo, tomato, onion, avocado, sour cream, and cilantro and serve.

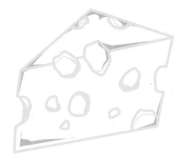

# *Aguacate Relleno* (Baked Avocado with Bacon and Cheese)

Life is better with avocados. I love how savory and smooth this recipe tastes and how it helps me stay full. As if that wasn't enough, the avocado is not only teeming with the good fat we need to fuel our body, it's also rich in vitamins and minerals and actually contains twice as much potassium as the sugar-charged banana.

**SERVES 2**
**PREP TIME:** 5 minutes
**COOK TIME:** 20 minutes

1 large avocado, halved and pitted (skin left on)
2 small eggs
Kosher salt and freshly ground black pepper to taste
2 slices bacon, chopped
2 tablespoons shredded mozzarella
2 teaspoons sliced fresh chives, for garnish

1. Preheat the oven to 425°F.
2. Place the avocado halves cut side up in two corners of a small baking dish (this prevents them from tipping over).
3. Crack an egg into each avocado half and season with salt and pepper.
4. Top with the bacon and mozzarella and bake until the eggs are set and the bacon is crisp, 15 to 20 minutes. Garnish with the chives and serve.

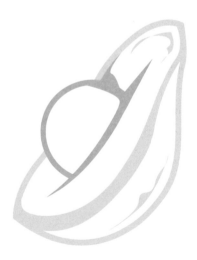

# Chi-Muffins (Tex-Mex Avocado Ham Eggs)

I'm always on the go, and there are mornings when all I have time to do is jump out of bed, get glammed up, and haul ass to my first meeting of the day. That's when these Chi-Muffins come in handy. I can make them the night before, then pop a couple in the microwave and have them in the car before applying my lipstick to finish my look of the day. If you have a hectic schedule, store the remaining muffins in the fridge and enjoy them the rest of the week as a quick-and-easy breakfast.

**MAKES 12 MUFFINS**
(2 or 3 per serving)
**PREP TIME:** 10 minutes
**COOK TIME:** 25 minutes

Cooking spray
5 large eggs
5 large egg whites
¼ cup unsweetened almond milk
4 tablespoons mild to medium salsa or pico de gallo
½ cup coarsely chopped ham (about 2 ounces)
1 teaspoon dried cilantro
½ teaspoon hot pepper flakes
¼ cup shredded cheddar cheese
1 teaspoon kosher salt
1 avocado, halved, pitted, peeled, and diced

1. Preheat the oven to 375°F. Spray a 12-cup muffin tin with cooking spray.
2. In a large mixing bowl, whisk together the eggs, egg whites, almond milk, salsa, ham, dried cilantro, hot pepper flakes, cheese, and salt.
3. Scoop ¼ cup of the mixture into each muffin cup.
4. Bake until a toothpick inserted in the center of a muffin comes out clean, about 25 minutes. Cool for 5 minutes in the pan, then turn the muffins out of the pan and serve topped with the avocado.

# Fajita Frittata

There's nothing like taking your basic frittata and spicing it up with Latin flavors. Add some Valentina hot sauce to the mix for that extra kick and you're good to go! Just make sure your hot sauce choice doesn't have any added sugar.

**SERVES 4**
**PREP TIME:** 10 minutes
**COOK TIME:** 30 minutes

6 slices bacon, cut into 1-inch lengths (about 5½ ounces)

6 ounces fresh spinach, coarsely chopped

¾ cup crumbled feta or Cotija cheese

¼ cup chopped green bell peppers

7 large eggs

¼ cup heavy cream

½ teaspoon kosher salt

½ teaspoon freshly ground black pepper

1. Preheat the oven to 350°F.
2. In a large, ovenproof, nonstick skillet, cook the bacon over medium heat until it has rendered its fat and is cooked through, about 4 minutes. Remove the bacon to a bowl, along with 1 tablespoon of the bacon fat. Leave the remaining fat in the skillet.
3. Add the spinach to the skillet and cook until wilted, about 2 minutes. Drain it well and squeeze dry.
4. Return the spinach to the skillet and spread it out, then scatter the bacon, cheese, and bell peppers over it.
5. In a large bowl, whisk together the eggs, cream, salt, and black pepper. Pour the egg mixture into the skillet and bake until the frittata is set and fluffy, about 20 minutes.

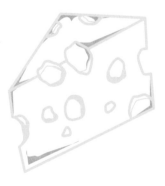

# Chi-Keto Horchata Smoothie

My grandma makes the best horchata in the world. The flavor in this smoothie brings me back to my *abuelita*'s kitchen and all the time I spent with her when I was around seven or eight. There was always a pot of *frijoles de la olla* on the stove, and her house smelled of that or Pine-Sol. I loved asking her if she would make me an *agua de horchata*, which was a total treat for me, and she'd always say yes. I enjoyed watching her put it together; I found it so intriguing that it was made out of rice. And it was so delicious. That's why drinking this keto-friendly version always makes me feel like a little girl, all fuzzy and whole inside.

**SERVES 1**

**PREP TIME:** 5 minutes

½ cup water

½ cup unsweetened coconut milk

½ cup blanched almonds

¼ cup egg white protein powder

1 tablespoon extra-virgin coconut butter

1 tablespoon ground chia seeds

1 teaspoon ground cinnamon

1 teaspoon pure vanilla extract

1 cup ice cubes

In a blender, puree all the ingredients until thick and smooth.

# Chilaquiles con Chicharrón and Avocado Crema

When I was about eight years old, I'd go visit my dad on the weekends, and he would make the best chilaquiles, nice and crispy. I love that this recipe maintains that crispiness and beautifully re-creates those flavors that just make me feel like I'm home.

**SERVES 2**
**PREP TIME:** 10 minutes
**COOK TIME:** 20 minutes

2 tablespoons avocado oil
4 ounces chicharrón
⅓ cup finely chopped red onion
¼ cup enchilada sauce
1 (4-ounce) can chopped green chiles
2 tablespoons chopped fresh cilantro
⅔ cup water
½ teaspoon kosher salt
¼ teaspoon freshly ground black pepper
4 large eggs, lightly beaten
Avocado Crema, *recipe follows*
1 tablespoon shredded Cotija cheese
2 radishes, thinly sliced

1. In a large skillet, heat the oil over medium heat. Add the chicharrón and cook, stirring frequently until crisp, about 4 minutes. With a slotted spoon transfer the chicharrón to a bowl and set aside.
2. Add the onion to the skillet and cook, stirring occasionally until crisp-tender, about 3 minutes. Add the enchilada sauce, green chiles, cilantro, and water and bring to a simmer. Cook, stirring occasionally until the sauce has thickened enough to coat the back of a spoon, about 7 minutes. Stir in the salt and pepper.
3. Stir the eggs into the skillet along with the chicharrón and cook, stirring occasionally, until the eggs are set, 2 to 3 minutes.
4. Pour the avocado crema over the chilaquiles and top with the cheese and radishes.

## Avocado Crema
**MAKES 1 CUP**

1 large avocado, halved, pitted, peeled, and cut into chunks
2 tablespoons Mexican crema
1 tablespoon fresh lime juice
2 to 3 tablespoons water
½ teaspoon kosher salt

In a blender, puree all the ingredients until smooth.

# Chocolate Blueberry Pancakes

Here's another recipe that reminds me of my weekends with my dad when I was a kid. If he wasn't making chilaquiles for us, he'd be mixing up some batter and making a stack of Mickey Mouse pancakes that made us oh so happy. You can never go wrong with pancakes, and this here feels like dessert for breakfast. Give me a little more of that keto-friendly syrup, please!

**MAKES 12 PANCAKES (2 per serving)**
**PREP TIME:** 10 minutes
**COOK TIME:** 15 minutes

4 ounces cream cheese, room temperature

2 tablespoons grass-fed butter, room temperature

4 large eggs

1 scoop carb-free chocolate protein powder (about ½ cup)

½ teaspoon vanilla extract

½ teaspoon ground cinnamon

Cooking spray

3 cups fresh blueberries

6 teaspoons sugar-free maple syrup

1. In a food processor, combine the cream cheese, butter, and eggs and process until smooth. Add the protein powder, vanilla, and cinnamon and pulse to combine.

2. Spray a small nonstick skillet with cooking spray and heat over medium heat. Pour 3 tablespoons of the batter into the pan and swirl the pan so the batter spreads out to make a thin pancake, 5 to 6 inches in diameter. Cook for about 30 seconds on each side, or until golden brown.

3. Top each serving with ½ cup blueberries and a teaspoon of sugar-free maple syrup.

# Blueberry Cheesecake Bar

When I'm in full PMS mode and cravings are kicking my behind, this is one of my favorite go-to breakfasts. It satisfies my sweet tooth and is easy to make. Bonus: you can refrigerate or freeze leftovers for the next time you are aching for a little something sweet. Added bonus: blueberries are low in sugar and high in vitamin C and antioxidants that will keep you healthy and glowing throughout the day.

**MAKES 9 SQUARES (2 per serving)**
**PREP TIME:** 10 minutes
**COOK TIME:** 25 minutes

Cooking spray
¾ cup organic coconut oil, melted
4 ounces cream cheese, room temperature, cut into cubes
4 tablespoons erythritol
½ teaspoon baking powder
Pinch of kosher salt
6 medium eggs
2 teaspoons vanilla extract
¼ cup frozen blueberries

1. Preheat the oven to 325°F. Spray an 8 × 8-inch baking dish with cooking spray.
2. In the bowl of an electric mixer with a paddle or a whisk attachment, beat the oil, cream cheese, erythritol, baking powder, and salt until well combined and smooth. Beat in the eggs and vanilla until well combined.
3. Pour the batter into the prepared baking dish and scatter the blueberries over the top; do not mix in the blueberries.
4. Bake until a toothpick inserted in the center comes out clean, 20 to 25 minutes. Cool completely in the pan before cutting into 9 squares. Serve from the pan. You can eat 1 or 2 squares per serving. Refrigerate or freeze any leftovers in an airtight container.

# Machaca con Huevos (Dried Beef with Eggs)

Growing up, I'd always heard that the best meat comes from Sonora, Mexico. I can vouch for that: the best *machaca* (dried beef) I've ever tried is the one from my great-grandma Nana Lola's hometown of Hermosillo in Sonora. When we'd pack up the car and take a drive down to visit her, she'd always serve up *machaca con huevos* with a side of flour tortillas for breakfast. This recipe takes me back to those trips, hanging out with Nana Lola and my *tíos* and rushing out to the backyard after breakfast with the sofa's foam cushions in hand, ready to start climbing up and sliding down the mountain. As the years went by and those trips became less frequent, my *abuelita* always made a point of bringing back a bag of *machaca* from her visits, and we'd have it every day until it was gone. Insert slurping noise here!

SERVES 1
PREP TIME: 10 minutes
COOK TIME: 20 minutes

1 tablespoon avocado oil
½ cup finely chopped yellow onion
1 cup dry beef (jerky), shredded (about 3 ounces)
1 medium tomato, coarsely chopped
2 serrano peppers, finely chopped (ribs and seeds removed for less heat, if desired)
2 large eggs, lightly beaten
2 tablespoons shredded cheddar cheese

1. In a large skillet, heat the oil over medium heat and cook the onion until crisp-tender, about 4 minutes. Stir in the beef and cook, stirring frequently until the beef starts to soften, about 4 minutes.

2. Lower the heat, stir in the tomato and serranos, and cook until slightly thickened, about 4 minutes.

3. Add the eggs and cheese and cook, stirring frequently, until the eggs are set but still soft, 4 to 5 minutes.

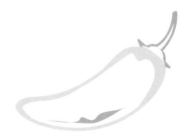

# Coconut Pancakes

You can never have enough of this breakfast. If you need a little extra sweet kick, top it with a handful of strawberries and some whipped cream and join me in saying: "Coco makes me loco!"

MAKES EIGHT 3- TO 4-INCH
  PANCAKES (2 per serving)
PREP TIME: 10 minutes
COOK TIME: 10 minutes

3 large eggs, separated

Pinch of kosher salt

6 tablespoons unsweetened coconut milk

3 tablespoons melted coconut oil, plus
  more as needed

¼ cup coconut flour

½ teaspoon baking powder

4 teaspoons sugar-free maple syrup

4 tablespoons unsweetened shredded
  coconut

1. In the bowl of an electric mixer with the whisk attachment, beat the egg whites and salt to soft peaks; set aside.

2. Whisk the coconut milk and 1 tablespoon of the coconut oil into the bowl with the yolks. Whisk in the coconut flour and baking powder until well combined and smooth.

3. With a rubber spatula, gently fold the egg whites into the yolk mixture. Let stand at room temperature until thickened, 2 to 3 minutes.

4. In a large nonstick skillet, heat the remaining 2 tablespoons coconut oil over medium-low heat. Drop the batter by 3 to 4 tablespoons into the pan and cook, working in batches, until the undersides are golden brown, about 2 minutes. Flip the pancakes over and cook 1 to 2 minutes longer, or until the undersides are golden brown. Add more oil if necessary to cook all the pancakes.

5. Top each serving with a teaspoon of the sugar-free maple syrup and 1 tablespoon of unsweetened shredded coconut.

# Ham and Cheese Omelet Stuffed in Bell Pepper

This is basically chile relleno's sister from another mister. Filled with its subtly sweet flavor, the bell pepper is a fantastic low-carb vegetable and a perfect match for this savory and cheesy egg mixture. It's a super-fulfilling way to start your day, especially after one of Sarah's workouts. Plus, it tastes great and helps you hit all your macros in one go.

SERVES 1
PREP TIME: 10 minutes
COOK TIME: 45 minutes

1 large bell pepper (red, green, or yellow)
2 small eggs
3 tablespoons heavy cream
¼ teaspoon kosher salt
¼ teaspoon freshly ground black pepper
3 slices ham, coarsely chopped
½ cup shredded mozzarella cheese
2 tablespoons finely chopped chives, plus more for garnish

1. Preheat the oven to 425°F.
2. Cut the top off the pepper and reserve. Cut out the ribs and seeds and discard. Cut a very thin slice off the bottom of the pepper so it stands upright and place the pepper and its top in a small baking dish and bake 6 minutes to soften slightly.
3. Meanwhile, in a small bowl, beat together the eggs, cream, salt, and black pepper. Stir in the ham, cheese, and chives.
4. Stand the pepper upright, pour in the egg mixture, and place the top on. Bake until the eggs are set, about 35 minutes. Garnish with chives.

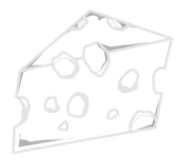

# Bacon Avocado Bomb

If you've been looking into keto, you've probably come across the phrase *fat bomb*. This is usually a bite-size piece of food that contains between 75 and 85 percent fat content. Most of the fat bombs out there are made with grass-fed butter, ghee, coconut oil, or cream cheese and tend to be on the sweet side. So I wanted to bring you a savory version. It will give you a great energy boost, perfect for when you have a long day ahead of you. Toss it on a slice of keto-friendly toast, add a spoonful of salsa, and you've got your version of a keto avocado toast.

**SERVES 2**
**PREP TIME:** 5 minutes
**COOK TIME:** 8 minutes

1 avocado, halved, pitted, and peeled
¼ cup shredded cheddar cheese
4 slices bacon

1. Heat the broiler on low with the rack 8 inches from the heat.
2. Fill one half of the avocado with the cheese, then top it with the other half. Wrap the bacon around the avocado and place it on a broiler pan.
3. Broil until the bacon is crisp, about 4 minutes. With tongs, carefully turn the avocado over and cook until the bacon is crisp all over, about 4 minutes longer. To serve, cut the avocado and halve lengthwise.

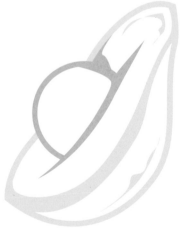

# Blueberry Chia Pudding

This pudding is super easy to prep the night before, making it another great breakfast when you are on the run. It's great if you're craving a sweet way to start your day, while also feeding your body with an explosion of good-for-you ingredients, like blueberries, almonds, and chia seeds, which are super rich in fiber and will help keep you fuller longer and get things moving!

**SERVES 1**
**PREP TIME:** 5 minutes
**SETTING TIME:** 4 hours to overnight

1 cup unsweetened coconut milk

½ cup frozen blueberries (defrosted) or fresh

2 tablespoons ground chia seeds

Handful of sliced almonds

1 teaspoon unsweetened shredded coconut

1 teaspoon unsweetened shaved dark chocolate

1. In a food processor or blender, puree the coconut milk, blueberries, and chia seeds until smooth. Transfer to a bowl and refrigerate until thick, at least 4 hours, but overnight is best.

2. Remove from the refrigerator and top with the almonds, coconut, and dark chocolate.

# Sausage Torta

This is an oh-so-savory and juicy meat-lover's delight. I love having this torta right after a high-intensity workout, because it helps satisfy the hunger that hits after leaving it all on the training floor. It's also perfect for those days when you need a little more food in your system, something that will keep you fuller longer, especially if you have back-to-back meetings and aren't sure when you'll be able to break for lunch. I give it an extra kick with my handy Valentina sauce and then I'm ready for what the day may bring. If you want to take it a step further, add a spoonful of salsa and a dollop of sour cream and do your happy dance.

**SERVES 1**
**PREP TIME:** 5 minutes
**COOK TIME:** 10 minutes

2 teaspoons olive oil

2 sausage patties (2 ounces each)

1 large egg

1 tablespoon cream cheese, at room temperature

1 tablespoon shredded sharp cheddar cheese

¼ teaspoon kosher salt

¼ to ½ teaspoon Tapatío hot sauce

1 teaspoon grass-fed butter

¼ medium avocado, peeled and sliced

1. In a small skillet, heat the oil over medium heat and cook the sausage patties until cooked through, about 2 minutes per side. Transfer to a serving plate. Set the skillet aside to be used to cook the egg mixture.

2. In a small bowl, lightly beat the egg and stir in the cream cheese, cheddar, salt, and Tapatío.

3. In the same skillet, melt the butter over low heat, add the egg mixture, and cook, stirring constantly, until the egg is set but still soft, about 4 minutes.

4. Top one sausage patty with the egg and avocado and place the second patty on top.

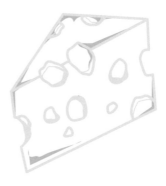

# Chi-Keto Pancakes

If you're more of a no-frills type of girl, who appreciates the simple things in life, then these pancakes are for you. No extras, just simple deliciousness to satisfy that pancake craving so you can get on with your day without ever feeling deprived.

**MAKES 4 PANCAKES** (2 per serving)
**PREP TIME:** 5 minutes
**COOK TIME:** 3 minutes

2 large eggs
2 ounces cream cheese, softened
¼ teaspoon ground cinnamon
½ teaspoon erythritol
½ teaspoon vanilla extract
1 teaspoon grass-fed butter, plus more as needed
Sugar-free maple syrup, for serving

1. In a food processor or blender, combine the eggs, cream cheese, cinnamon, erythritol, and vanilla and process until smooth. Set aside and let the batter rest for a couple of minutes.

2. In a small nonstick skillet, heat the butter over medium-low heat until melted. Drop 2 teaspoonfuls of the batter into the pan and swirl the pan so the batter covers the bottom. Cook until bubbles appear on the surface and the underside is lightly browned, about 20 seconds. Carefully flip the pancake over and cook about 5 seconds longer until set. Transfer to a plate and continue with the remaining batter, adding more butter if necessary.

3. Serve the pancakes with sugar-free maple syrup or whipped cream, if desired.

# Portobello Egg Toast

I love mushrooms! And this particular recipe makes me feel like I'm eating a breakfast pizza. The juicy portobello makes a great meat substitute (for all the veggie lovers in the house!), is low in calories, and gives you a wonderful boost of selenium and copper. It's also a great source of potassium, which is especially important now that bananas aren't part of your everyday diet.

**SERVES 2**
**PREP TIME:** 7 minutes
**COOK TIME:** 20 minutes

2 large portobello mushrooms (4½ inches in diameter), stems removed
Cooking spray
1 teaspoon kosher salt
½ teaspoon freshly ground black pepper
½ teaspoon garlic powder
2 medium eggs
¼ cup grated Parmesan cheese
2 tablespoons chopped parsley, for garnish

1. Preheat the oven 400°F.
2. With a spoon, scrape out the gills from the mushrooms and discard. Spray the mushroom caps on both sides with cooking spray and season with the salt, pepper, and garlic powder. Place the caps stemmed side up on a small rimmed sheet pan and bake until tender, about 4 minutes. Remove the caps to a plate and place stemmed side down to drain.
3. Spray two 6-ounce ramekins or custard cups with cooking spray and push the mushroom caps stemmed side up into the ramekins. Crack an egg into each mushroom cap and top with the Parmesan. Place the ramekins on the rimmed sheet pan and bake until the eggs are set, about 10 minutes. Garnish with the parsley to serve.

# Cheesy Turkey Egg Tacos

I am a taco fiend! I can eat breakfast tacos all day every day. Knowing that I can enjoy the crunch of this cheesy taco melded with my favorite flavors while on keto just makes me smile. I love this recipe so much that sometimes I make it for dinner too, especially if I'm craving this type of crispy delight.

**SERVES 3**
**PREP TIME:** 10 minutes
**COOK TIME:** 15 minutes

1 cup shredded low-moisture mozzarella cheese

1 tablespoon grass-fed butter

3 large eggs, lightly beaten

2 slices cooked turkey breast, diced (about 3 ounces)

¼ cup shredded cheddar cheese

¼ teaspoon kosher salt

¼ teaspoon freshly ground black pepper

½ small avocado, pitted, peeled, and diced

1. Preheat the oven to 350°F. Line a rimmed sheet pan with parchment paper.
2. Drop three ⅓-cup mounds of mozzarella onto the prepared sheet pan, spacing them several inches apart and flattening them slightly. Bake until the cheese has melted and the edges have browned slightly, 8 to 10 minutes. Remove from the oven and let stand 2 to 3 minutes until set but still pliable.
3. Place a long wooden spoon with a round handle over a large bowl. Drape the slightly cooled mozzarella over the wooden spoon until firm to make the taco shells.
4. In a large nonstick skillet, heat the butter over medium-low heat. Add the eggs, turkey, cheese, salt, and pepper and cook, stirring frequently, until the eggs are set but still soft, about 4 minutes.
5. Spoon one-third of the scrambled egg mixture into each shell and top with the avocado.

# Crispy Cinnamon Almond Waffles

When I'm yearning for the classic French toast or waffles that my girlfriends order during Sunday brunch, I turn to these babies. They're so yummy that they really help you feel like you're not missing out. Plus, they taste like Christmas in your mouth.

**SERVES 2**
**PREP TIME:** 5 minutes
**COOK TIME:** 5 minutes

½ cup superfine almond flour
½ teaspoon erythritol
¼ teaspoon kosher salt
¼ teaspoon baking soda
¼ teaspoon baking powder
¼ teaspoon ground cinnamon
⅛ teaspoon grated nutmeg
⅛ teaspoon ground cloves
2 large eggs, separated
1 teaspoon vanilla extract
2 tablespoons melted vanilla ghee
Sugar-free maple syrup, for serving
Ground cinnamon, for serving

1. In a medium bowl, whisk together the almond flour, erythritol, salt, baking soda, baking powder, cinnamon, nutmeg, and cloves.
2. In the bowl of an electric mixer fitted with the whisk attachment, beat the egg whites to soft peaks. Set aside.
3. In a separate bowl, combine the yolks, vanilla, and ghee and stir into the almond flour mixture.
4. With a rubber spatula, gently fold the egg whites into the almond flour mixture.
5. Cook the batter in a waffle maker following the manufacturer's directions. Top the waffles with sugar-free maple syrup and a sprinkle of cinnamon.

# Pumpkin Spice Coffee Smoothie

Give up pumpkin spice in the fall? Why? Instead of gazing nostalgically at everyone around you with their pumpkin-spiced fill-in-the-blank, make this smoothie and join the pumpkin-loving crowd. Soon enough, your friends will be asking for the recipe to enjoy this creamy cup of goodness.

**SERVES 2**
**PREP TIME:** 5 minutes

½ cup unsweetened coconut milk
½ cup unsweetened coconut cream
1 tablespoon unsweetened pumpkin puree
1 tablespoon hemp seeds
1½ teaspoons pumpkin pie spice
1 teaspoon loose chai tea
1 teaspoon vanilla extract
1 teaspoon (or more if you wish) instant coffee
½ cup ice water
½ avocado, pitted, peeled and cut into chunks
Ice cubes, if desired

In a blender, puree all the ingredients except the avocado until smooth. Add the avocado and ice cubes, if desired, and puree until smooth. Divide between 2 glasses.

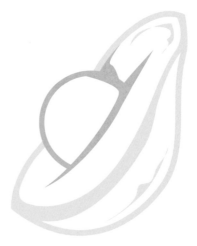

# Chocolate Green Creamy Smoothie

The hemp seeds and avocado give this smoothie a rich and creamy texture that's to die for, while the dark leafy greens tick off the "Eat Yo' Veggies" list and fuel your body with nutritious goodness. To top it off, the flavor of the cacao powder makes me feel like I'm a kid in an ice cream parlor, slurping on a chocolate milkshake. This is another great breakfast for when you're PMSing or needing to satisfy your sweet tooth.

**SERVES 2**
**PREP TIME:** 5 minutes

1¼ cups filtered water
½ avocado, pitted, peeled and cut into
  chunks
½ cucumber, peeled, seeded, and sliced
1 cup dark leafy greens
2 tablespoons parsley leaves
2 tablespoons hemp seeds
1 tablespoon raw coconut butter
2½ tablespoons lemon juice
1 teaspoon raw unsweetened cacao powder
¼ teaspoon ground turmeric
2 dandelion leaves, if desired

In a blender, combine all the ingredients and puree until smooth. Divide between 2 glasses.

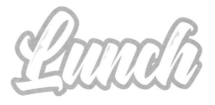

# Lunch

*Eat lunch so you don't become hangry. Lunch is here to help us stay energized, crush the afternoon meetings, and power through the rest of the day like boss bees building their empires and shutting shit down. I can't get enough of the Chicken Chipotle Casserole (page 94) bursting with homey flavors. And the Chile Relleno with Ground Chicken (page 98) . . . with lots of hot sauce, of course!*

## Chingona Tip

When I started my Chi-Keto journey, I did my best to stay away from any type of fruit juices or sugary sodas. If you're craving them hard, go for a sugar-free flavored sparkling water. Just add a slice of lime or lemon to the mix and it's almost like you're having the real thing!

# Aguachile

*¡Ay, qué rico!* The *aguachile* (a name that literally means *chile water*) is said to come from Sinaloa, Mexico, and is considered a type of Mexican ceviche. Pair this refreshing recipe with my keto-friendly Michelada (page 146) and you've got the perfect Sunday Funday meal. If you like, replace the Mozzarella Tostadas (page 80) with a cup of chopped iceberg lettuce and turn this dish into an aguachile salad!

**SERVES 2**
**PREP TIME:** 20 minutes
**MARINATING TIME:** 1½ to 2 hours
**COOK TIME:** 10 minutes

1 pound large shrimp (about 18), peeled and deveined
1 cup fresh lime juice
Kosher salt to taste
¼ cup olive oil
4 serrano peppers, finely chopped (ribs and seeds removed for less heat, if desired)
¼ cup cold water
1 medium cucumber, peeled and thinly sliced
1 medium red onion, halved and thinly sliced
1 avocado, halved, pitted, peeled, and diced, for garnish
⅓ cup finely chopped cilantro, for garnish
Mozzarella Tostadas (page 80)

1. In a large bowl, toss the shrimp with ½ cup of the lime juice and ½ teaspoon kosher salt. Cover and refrigerate 1½ to 2 hours (longer marinating will make the shrimp tough).

2. In a blender, combine the remaining ½ cup lime juice, the olive oil, serrano peppers, and water and blend until thick. Season with salt.

3. Divide the cucumber and onion between two plates. Top with the shrimp, drizzle with the sauce, and garnish with the avocado and cilantro. Serve with mozzarella tostadas.

## Mozzarella Tostadas

I can't get enough of how crunchy and savory these tostadas are. Keep this recipe handy because you'll soon be using it for so much more, like re-creating Mexican tostadas. I think I know what I'm making tonight!

**MAKES 4 TOSTADAS (2 per serving)**

1 cup shredded mozzarella

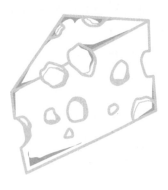

1. Preheat the oven to 350°F. Line a rimmed sheet pan with parchment paper.
2. Make 4 equal mounds of cheese on the prepared baking sheet and flatten them slightly. Bake until melted and crisp, 8 to 12 minutes.
3. Cool for 5 minutes before serving.

# *Chile Gordo* (Chicken-and-Cheese-Stuffed Poblano Peppers)

There ain't nothin' *gordo* about this chile! Nothing but deliciousness. I mean, come on, how can we go wrong with a chicken, cheese, and poblano pepper combo topped with sour cream . . . and it's keto-friendly! Chile Gordo, where have you been all my life?

**SERVES 4**
**PREP TIME:** 10 minutes
**COOK TIME:** 30 minutes

½ cup sour cream, plus more for serving

⅓ cup pico de gallo

1 cup shredded cheddar cheese

1 cup shredded queso blanco

¼ cup thinly sliced scallions, plus more for serving

2 tablespoons chopped cilantro, plus more for serving

2 jalapeño or serrano peppers, finely chopped (ribs and seeds removed for less heat, if desired)

4 cups cubed cooked chicken (about 20 ounces)

4 medium poblano peppers (5 ounces each)

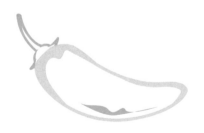

1. In a large bowl, combine the sour cream, pico de gallo, ¾ cup of the cheddar, ¾ cup of the queso blanco, the scallions, cilantro, and jalapeños. Add the chicken, stir to combine, and refrigerate.

2. Heat the broiler on low with the rack 6 inches from the heat.

3. Place the poblanos on a broiler pan or sheet pan and broil, turning them as the skin blackens, about 10 minutes total. Transfer to a plate and let stand for 10 minutes. When cool enough to handle, use your fingers to peel the skin, cut the peppers in half, and gently remove the seeds.

4. Preheat the oven to 350°F.

5. Spoon about ¾ cup of the chicken mixture onto each pepper half and top with the remaining halves. Place on a rimmed sheet pan and bake for 10 minutes. Scatter the remaining cheddar and queso blanco over the peppers and bake until the filling is piping hot and the cheese has melted, about 10 minutes more. Serve with sour cream, scallions, and cilantro.

# À la Chi-Taco Salad (Chicken Taco Salad with Chipotle Ranch Dressing)

One of the things I love the most about my keto-friendly lifestyle is that I can still enjoy the flavors I grew up with. We're striking the balance between food that will get our health and body on the path to fabulousness and recipes that taste effing amazing. The combination of the taco-seasoned chicken, Cotija cheese, cilantro, avocado, and chipotle dressing spice up this salad and make it an all-day fiesta in my mouth.

**SERVES 2**
**PREP TIME:** 20 minutes
**COOK TIME:** 10 minutes

¼ cup olive oil
½ small yellow onion, chopped
2 boneless, skinless chicken breasts (6 ounces each), cut into 1-inch chunks
2 tablespoons taco seasoning
1 large head romaine lettuce, coarsely chopped
2 small Roma (plum) tomatoes, diced
1 cup shredded Cotija cheese
2 avocados, halved, pitted, peeled, and diced
2 scallions, thinly sliced
½ cup fresh cilantro leaves
Chipotle Ranch Dressing (page 83)

1. In a large nonstick skillet, heat the oil over medium-low heat. Add the onion and cook, stirring occasionally, until crisp-tender, about 3 minutes. Add the chicken, sprinkle the taco seasoning over, and cook, stirring occasionally, until the chicken is cooked through, about 4 minutes.

2. In a large bowl, layer the lettuce, chicken and any juices, tomatoes, cheese, avocados, scallions, and cilantro. Drizzle with 3 to 4 tablespoons of the dressing, toss to combine, and serve.

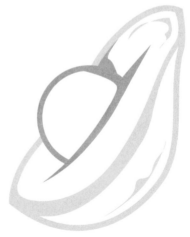

# Chipotle Ranch Dressing

**MAKES ABOUT 1⅓ CUPS**

½ cup mayonnaise

½ cup sour cream

¼ cup heavy cream

1 canned chipotle pepper in adobo

2 tablespoons fresh parsley

1 tablespoon cilantro leaves

1 tablespoon fresh lime juice

1 teaspoon apple cider vinegar

2 teaspoons smoked paprika

1 teaspoon ground cumin

1 teaspoon onion powder

⅛ teaspoon garlic powder

In a blender or food processor, puree all the ingredients until smooth.

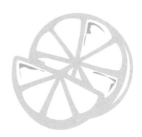

# *Not Your Basic Chick* (Protein-Style Parmesan Cheese Chicken Burger Verde)

One of my favorite pre-Chi-Keto meals were chicken burgers. I thought I'd have to give them up, but by simply swapping the carb-loaded buns with crispy butter lettuce leaves, we were able to re-create a healthy alternative to the chicken burgers I've always loved! This dish will give you a boost of good fats and proteins and help you feel like you're not missing out. Season it with your favorite keto-friendly sauce (meaning sugar-free, *chula*!) and let that beautiful smile shine through each bite.

**SERVES 4**
**PREP TIME:** 10 minutes
**COOK TIME:** 10 minutes

1 pound ground chicken
1 cup grated Parmesan cheese
½ cup finely chopped yellow onion
½ cup chopped fresh parsley
1 jalapeño, finely chopped (ribs and seeds removed for less heat, if desired)
1 clove garlic, finely chopped
¾ teaspoon kosher salt
1 teaspoon paprika
1 tablespoon olive oil
8 butter lettuce leaves

1. In a large bowl, combine the chicken, Parmesan, onion, parsley, jalapeño, garlic, salt, and paprika. Shape into eight 3 × ½-inch patties.
2. In a large nonstick skillet, heat the oil over medium heat. Add the patties and cook until just cooked through, about 3 minutes per side.
3. Divide the patties and lettuce among four plates. Serve each with your choice of toppings and 1 teaspoon of your favorite keto-friendly sauce.

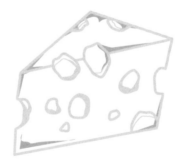

# Chi-Keto Burgers (Portobello Bun Turkey Cheeseburgers with Pico de Gallo)

When I think of ground turkey, I think of the dry diet food that you order from meal-prep companies. But this couldn't be further from that image. It's mouthwatering and juicy, and the spices and pico de gallo give it an awesome kick of flavor. It's perfect for when you're craving a cheeseburger or need a lunch that will keep you full and satisfied throughout the rest of your day.

**SERVES 1**
**PREP TIME:** 10 minutes
**COOK TIME:** 20 minutes

4 teaspoons olive oil
1 clove garlic, finely chopped
1 teaspoon dried oregano
½ teaspoon kosher salt
1⅛ teaspoons freshly ground black pepper
2 portobello mushroom caps (4½ inches in diameter), stemmed
6 ounces (85% lean) ground turkey
¼ cup shredded Colby Jack cheese
1 tablespoon Dijon mustard
½ jalapeño, finely chopped (ribs and seeds removed for less heat, if desired)
1 tablespoon pico de gallo
Small handful of arugula

1. In a small bowl, combine 2 teaspoons of the oil, the garlic, oregano, ¼ teaspoon of the salt, and ⅛ of the teaspoon pepper.
2. With a spoon, scrape out the gills of the mushrooms. Brush the scraped sides with the olive oil mixture.
3. In a large nonstick skillet, heat 1 teaspoon of the remaining oil over medium-low heat. Place the mushrooms scraped side up in the skillet, cover, and cook until tender, about 8 minutes. Transfer the mushrooms scraped side down to a plate to drain.
4. In a small bowl, combine the turkey, cheese, Dijon, jalapeño, and the remaining 1 teaspoon pepper and ¼ teaspoon salt. Shape into a ½-inch-thick patty.
5. In a small nonstick skillet, heat the remaining 1 teaspoon oil over medium heat and cook the patty for about 5 minutes per side until cooked through. Top one portobello cap scraped side up with the patty, pico de gallo, and some arugula. Top with the second portobello cap scraped side down.

# Carnitas with Jalapeño Poppers (Mexican Pulled Pork with Stuffed Peppers)

Carnitas, extra crispy, please! Paired with the melt-in-your-mouth jalapeño poppers, um, I want one now. As my dad used to say, *Una buena mexicana tiene que saber comer chiles*, (a good Mexican has to know how to eat chiles). He gave me my first jalapeño when I was about five years old and taught me how to bite into it and withstand the heat. And that's now one of my favorite things to do. That's why I love jalapeños, Valentina and Tapatío sauces, and any type of chile. When I walk into a restaurant, I'm the one ordering *chiles toreados* or asking for their house-made salsa. I need a spicy kick in my meal to make it feel complete, which is why this recipe speaks to my heart. Yeah, I'm the girl who carries a hot sauce bottle in her purse on vacation or in case of emergencies. I just can't live without my chile!

**SERVES 6**
**PREP TIME:** 20 minutes
**COOK TIME:** 2 hours

2 tablespoons olive oil
2½ teaspoons kosher salt
1 teaspoon freshly ground black pepper
2 pounds boneless pork shoulder, cut into 4 large chunks
1 large yellow onion, coarsely chopped
5 cloves garlic, finely chopped
2 jalapeños, seeded and finely chopped
1 navel orange, halved
2 tablespoons fresh lime juice
2 teaspoons paprika
2 teaspoons ground cumin
1½ teaspoons ground coriander
Jalapeño Poppers (page 87)

1. Preheat the oven to 325°F.
2. In a large skillet, heat the oil over medium heat. Rub the salt and pepper into the pork and cook, working in batches if necessary, until richly browned, about 5 minutes per side. With a slotted spoon, transfer the meat to a Dutch oven.
3. Add the onion, garlic, and jalapeños to the skillet and cook, stirring frequently until the onion is tender, about 7 minutes. Transfer to the Dutch oven with the meat. Add 1 cup of water to the skillet, scrape up any of the browned bits, and pour into the Dutch oven. Squeeze the juice of the orange halves into the skillet, then add the whole orange along with the lime juice, paprika, cumin, and coriander. Bring to a boil, cover, and transfer to the Dutch oven.
4. Bake until the meat is very tender, about 1½ hours, then shred the pork using two forks and serve with jalapeño poppers.

## Jalapeño Poppers

**MAKES 6 POPPERS**
**PREP TIME:** 10 minutes
**COOK TIME:** 20 minutes

3 ounces cream cheese, softened
¼ cup shredded cheddar cheese
¼ cup sliced scallions
1 tablespoon finely chopped cilantro
2 cloves garlic, finely chopped
6 medium jalapeño peppers, halved
  lengthwise and seeds removed

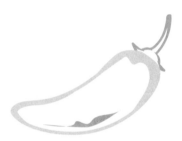

1. Preheat the oven to 400°F. Line a rimmed sheet pan with parchment paper or foil.
2. In a small bowl, mash together the cream cheese, cheddar, scallions, cilantro, and garlic. (Soften the cream cheese in the microwave if it is too hard.) With a spoon, divide the cheese mixture among the jalapeño halves, sandwich the halves back together, and transfer to the prepared sheet pan, spacing them apart.
3. Bake until the peppers are soft, about 20 minutes.

# Steak Fajita Salad with Cilantro Lime Dressing

You can never go wrong with a plate of fajitas. Both real and wannabe Mexican restaurants have this keto-friendly dish on their menus (say no to the tortillas, though!), and it's also so easy to make at home. It was actually one of the first main dishes I learned how to cook. I used to make fajitas for my siblings all the time to make sure they were eating their veggies and their protein. It was an easy go-to meal, although they always gave me crap about it because I made it so often. The savory flavors in this recipe topped with that amazing cilantro lime dressing is everything!

**SERVES 1**
**PREP TIME:** 10 minutes
**COOK TIME:** 10 minutes

1½ tablespoons fresh lime juice

6 teaspoons olive oil

1 teaspoon dried oregano

1 teaspoon garlic powder

½ teaspoon onion powder

½ teaspoon ground cumin

½ teaspoon chili powder

5 ounces flank steak, sliced ¼ inch thick across the grain

½ medium yellow onion, thinly sliced

½ red bell pepper, thinly sliced

½ orange bell pepper, thinly sliced

½ green bell pepper, thinly sliced

2 cups chopped romaine lettuce

Cilantro Lime Dressing (page 89)

1. In a small bowl, whisk together the lime juice, 1 teaspoon of the oil, the oregano, garlic powder, onion powder, cumin, and chili powder. Add the steak, tossing to coat.

2. In a large nonstick skillet, heat 3 teaspoons of the remaining oil over medium-high heat and cook the steak, turning the slices midway, about 1 minute total for medium. Remove to a bowl.

3. Add the remaining 2 teaspoons oil, the onion, and bell peppers to the skillet and cook over medium heat, stirring frequently, until the peppers are crisp-tender, about 4 minutes. Add to the bowl with the steak.

4. In a medium bowl, toss together the lettuce, steak, vegetables, and 2 tablespoons of dressing.

## Cilantro Lime Dressing
**MAKES ABOUT 1 CUP**

1 cup fresh cilantro
½ cup full-fat sour cream
¼ cup olive oil
3 tablespoons fresh lime juice
1 tablespoon plain Greek yogurt
1 teaspoon apple cider vinegar
½ clove garlic
Kosher salt and freshly ground black
   pepper to taste

In a food processor or blender, combine all the ingredients and blend until smooth. Season with salt and pepper.

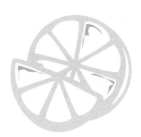

# Chicken Tortilla Soup

Any type of soup brings joy to my heart when I'm feeling sad or sick or anything—I honestly don't need an excuse to have *sopa*. But chicken tortilla soup is like chicken noodle soup for the soul *a la mexicana*. It automatically brings to mind my home and fills me with a sense of comfort and warmth.

SERVES 4
PREP TIME: 15 minutes
COOK TIME: 25 minutes

1 tablespoon olive oil

½ medium yellow onion, finely chopped

2 cloves garlic, finely chopped

1½ cups coarsely chopped zucchini (from an 8-ounce zucchini)

½ medium red bell pepper, diced

2 chipotle peppers in adobo, finely chopped (about 2 tablespoons)

¾ teaspoon chili powder

1 teaspoon dried oregano

¾ teaspoon kosher salt

4 cups chicken broth

2 small Roma (plum) tomatoes, diced

1 (4-ounce) can chopped green chiles

2 cups shredded cooked chicken breast (about 10 ounces cooked)

1 avocado, halved, pitted, peeled, and diced

½ cup shredded Monterey Jack cheese

½ cup chopped cilantro

1 tablespoon fresh lime juice

*Toppings*

Sour cream

Sliced radishes

Lime wedges

Handful keto Moon cheese

1. In a large saucepan or Dutch oven, heat the oil over medium heat. Add the onion and garlic and cook until the onion is crisp-tender, about 4 minutes.

2. Add the zucchini, bell pepper, chipotle peppers, chili powder, oregano, and salt and cook, stirring frequently, until the bell pepper is crisp-tender, about 5 minutes.

3. Add the broth, tomatoes, and green chiles, partially cover, and simmer for 15 minutes. Stir in the chicken, avocado, cheese, cilantro, and lime juice and serve with your choice of toppings.

# Prosciutto Arugula Pizza

Many times, when you ask someone what their ultimate comfort food is, you'll notice that a lot of them will blurt out, "Pizza!" without giving it a second thought. So adopting a keto-friendly lifestyle for pizza lovers may sound daunting. But Chi-Keto's got your back. You not only can have your favorite slice on your indulgence day, you can also enjoy this pizza alternative that will help you satisfy that craving any day of the week.

**SERVES 2, MAKES 1 LARGE PIE**
**PREP TIME:** 15 minutes
**COOK TIME:** 45 minutes

*For the crust* (you can also use a store-bought, ready-made, low-carb cauliflower crust)
Cooking spray
1 head cauliflower (about 2 pounds), stalk removed, cut into florets
½ cup shredded mozzarella
¼ cup grated Parmesan
½ teaspoon dried oregano
½ teaspoon kosher salt
¼ teaspoon garlic powder
2 large eggs, lightly beaten

*For the topping*
Pesto (page 92)
4 ounces mozzarella cheese, thinly sliced
3 ounces nitrate-free prosciutto, thinly sliced
2 cups arugula
2 teaspoons fresh lemon juice
1 tablespoon olive oil

1. *For the crust:* Preheat the oven to 400°F. Spray a rimmed baking sheet with cooking spray.

2. In a food processor, pulse the cauliflower until finely ground.

3. Place the cauliflower, working in batches if necessary, in a steamer basket set over a pan of simmering water and cook until tender, about 4 minutes. If wet, place the cauliflower in a kitchen towel and squeeze dry. Let cool completely, transfer to a bowl, and add the mozzarella, Parmesan, oregano, salt, garlic powder, and eggs and mix until well combined.

4. Transfer the mixture to the prepared baking sheet and spread it out to a large round or rectangle ¼ inch thick. Bake until crisp and brown, about 30 minutes. Cool for 10 minutes.

5. *For the topping*: Spread the pesto over the crust. Top with the mozzarella and prosciutto and bake for 5 to 7 minutes, or until the cheese has melted.

6. In a small bowl, mix together the arugula, lemon juice, and olive oil. Scatter it over the pizza and serve.

## Pesto

MAKES ABOUT 1¼ CUPS

2 cups fresh basil
2 tablespoons pine nuts
2 cloves garlic
½ cup extra-virgin olive oil
½ cup grated Parmesan cheese
½ teaspoon kosher salt

In a food processor or blender, puree all the ingredients until smooth.

# Ground Turkey Stuffed Avocados

Creamy avocados stuffed with turkey and cheese already sound delicious, but what takes this dish to another level is that spicy tomatillo-pasilla sauce. I think it's clear I like to spice things up, and this is one hot and tempting sauce that brings this dish home. But don't stop here! Double up the sauce recipe and store the extra batch in your fridge, so it's ready to elevate any other meal that you feel may need an extra kick of *sabor*.

**SERVES 2**
**PREP TIME:** 10 minutes
**COOK TIME:** 15 minutes

2 tablespoons olive oil
¾ cup diced white onion
½ pound (85% lean) ground turkey
½ cup chopped cilantro
Tomatillo-Pasilla Sauce, *recipe follows*
Kosher salt to taste
2 avocados, halved, pitted, and peeled
2 tablespoons sour cream
2 tablespoons shredded Mexican cheese blend
2 teaspoons thinly sliced scallions

1. In a large skillet, heat the oil over medium heat. Add the onion and cook, stirring frequently, until tender, about 7 minutes. Add the turkey and cook, breaking the meat apart with a spatula until cooked through, about 5 minutes. Add the cilantro, stir in half the sauce, and add salt; simmer for 1 minute.

2. Divide the turkey mixture among the 4 avocado halves and top with the sour cream, cheese, scallions, and remaining sauce, if desired.

## Tomatillo-Pasilla Sauce
**MAKES 1½ CUPS**

2 to 3 pasilla chiles, depending upon desired degree of heat
10 soft tomatillos
2 cloves garlic, finely chopped
Kosher salt to taste

1. On a grill or in a small skillet, toast the pasilla chiles over medium heat for 2 minutes.

2. Transfer the chiles to a bowl of warm water and let them stand until softened, about 10 minutes. Remove the seeds and ribs and transfer the chiles to a food processor or blender along with the tomatillos, garlic, and salt and puree until smooth. Set aside.

# Chicken Chipotle Casserole

This is what I turn to when I'm craving enchiladas. When I hit my teens, my mom was the one who passed down her enchilada recipe to me. She showed me how to put the tortilla in the oil, then dip it in the red sauce, and patiently went through each of the following steps until I became an expert too. Once I had the method down, I started making it for my siblings, and it quickly became one of our long-time favorites when eating as a family. When I make this particular keto-friendly recipe, serve it, and take a bite, it also reminds me of lasagna, another dish that I adore. So it's kind of like the best of both worlds.

**SERVES 4**
**PREP TIME:** 15 minutes
**COOK TIME:** 40 minutes

Cooking spray
1 tablespoon olive oil
½ medium white onion, finely chopped
2 jalapeños, 1 coarsely chopped and 1 sliced (ribs and seeds removed for less heat, if desired)
2 chipotle peppers in adobo, chopped
4 ounces cream cheese, softened
¼ cup heavy cream
1 cup red enchilada sauce
1 pound boneless, skinless chicken thighs, cooked and shredded (about 3 cups)
2 low-carb tortillas
1 cup shredded cheddar cheese
Fresh cilantro, for garnish

1. Preheat the oven to 375°F. Spray a 9 × 9-inch baking dish with cooking spray.
2. In a large skillet, heat the oil over medium heat. Add the onion, chopped jalapeño, and chipotle peppers and cook, stirring frequently, until the onion is tender, about 5 minutes.
3. Add the cream cheese and heavy cream and cook, stirring occasionally, until the cream cheese has melted, about 1 minute. Stir in the enchilada sauce and shredded chicken and mix well.
4. Place the tortillas side by side in the prepared baking dish and spoon the chicken mixture over, spreading it evenly. Scatter the cheese over and top with the jalapeño slices.
5. Cover with foil and bake for 15 minutes. Uncover and bake until the cheese has melted and the dish is piping hot, about 15 minutes more. Garnish with cilantro and serve.

# Pollo en Mole Verde with Hemp Seed Rice

When I hear mole, I immediately think of my *abuelita*. She makes the best mole, hands down, and she makes it from scratch. Her mole is never too light or too dark; it's always just right. And to this day, if I ask her, she'll make it for me, and I'm immediately in heaven. My mom would also make her version of mole, but she'd turn to a jar of Doña María Mole for help. What I loved most about those meals was grabbing the empty Doña María jar and letting it sit in warm water while we ate so that I could easily peel off the label later. Then I'd use it the next day for my chocolate milk; it just made it extra special. We'd also use my Doña María jar collection to drink Kool-Aid or store salsa. They were like our very own set of mason jars. I love this particular mole recipe because it's not too sweet, it has a good amount of spice to it, it's easy to make, and it tastes like home.

**SERVES 4**
**PREP TIME:** 15 minutes
**COOK TIME:** 45 minutes

4 chicken legs (drumsticks and thighs; about 2¾ pounds)

1 large yellow onion, halved

5 cloves garlic

2¾ teaspoons kosher salt

½ cup coarsely chopped fresh tomatillos (about 3 ounces)

2 celery stalks, chopped (about ½ cup)

½ cup cilantro sprigs

3 tablespoons hulled pumpkin seeds

2 to 3 serrano peppers, seeded and coarsely chopped

1 tablespoon olive oil

6 tender nopales, cleaned, cut into thin strips, and cooked*

2 tablespoons grass-fed butter

4 medium mushrooms, coarsely chopped

1 cup hemp seeds

¼ cup chicken broth

¼ cup heavy cream

½ teaspoon garlic powder

¼ teaspoon dried parsley

⅛ teaspoon freshly ground black pepper

* See Costillas de Puerco en Adobo con Ensalada de Nopales (page 127) for directions on cleaning and cooking nopales.

1. In a large saucepan, bring the chicken, half the onion, 4 cloves of the garlic, 2 teaspoons of the salt, and 4 cups of water to a boil. Reduce to a simmer, skim any foam that rises to the top, cover, and cook until the chicken is cooked through, about 30 minutes.
2. Meanwhile, in a blender, puree the tomatillos, celery, cilantro, pumpkin seeds, serranos, ½ teaspoon of the remaining salt, the remaining onion half, the remaining clove of garlic, and ½ cup of the chicken cooking liquid until smooth.
3. In a large skillet, heat the oil over medium heat and bring the tomatillo sauce to a simmer. Add the chicken and nopales. Cover and simmer until the nopales and chicken are heated through, 5 to 7 minutes.
4. Meanwhile, in a medium skillet, melt the butter over medium heat. Add the mushrooms and cook, stirring occasionally, until tender, about 4 minutes.
5. Add the hemp seeds, chicken broth, cream, garlic powder, dried parsley, the remaining ¼ teaspoon salt, and the black pepper, reduce the heat to low, and cook until the liquid has been absorbed, about 5 minutes. Serve hot.

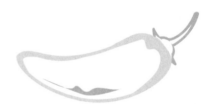

# Pechuga de Pollo en Salsa de Queso y Espinaca
## (Chicken Breast in Cheese and Spinach Sauce)

The creaminess of this sauce combined with the spinach and chicken makes me feel like I'm having guilt-free chicken Alfredo. And without the pasta, there's no afternoon slump to slow me down. It also brings me back to when I was a little girl and my *abuelita* would tell me that if I wanted to be as strong as Popeye, I had to have my spinach. She knew how to get to me because I thought Popeye was the bomb, and spinach still remains one of my all-time favorite vegetables.

**SERVES 4**
**PREP TIME:** 15 minutes
**COOK TIME:** 25 minutes

Olive oil
4 boneless, skinless chicken breasts (6 ounces each)
1 teaspoon paprika
1 teaspoon kosher salt
¼ teaspoon garlic powder
¼ teaspoon onion powder
4 ounces cream cheese, softened and cubed
½ cup grated Parmesan
2 tablespoons mayonnaise
1½ cups baby spinach, chopped (about 1¾ ounces)
1 teaspoon finely chopped garlic
½ teaspoon red chili pepper flakes

1. Preheat the oven to 375°F. Lightly oil a large baking dish.

2. Place the chicken on a cutting board and, with a chef's knife, cut into the thickest part, making a slit about 3 inches long. Wiggle the knife to cut about three-quarters of the way into the chicken without cutting through to the other side.

3. In a small bowl, combine the paprika, ¾ teaspoon of the salt, the garlic powder, and the onion powder and sprinkle the mixture over both sides of the chicken.

4. In a medium bowl, stir together the cream cheese, Parmesan, mayonnaise, spinach, garlic, pepper flakes, and the remaining ¼ teaspoon salt until smooth.

5. Fill a pastry bag without a tip with the spinach mixture and pipe it into the chicken pockets. Drizzle a little oil over the chicken. Bake until cooked through, about 25 minutes. Serve with the pan juices spooned over.

# Chile Relleno with Ground Chicken

Since this takes a little bit longer to prepare, I suggest using your time wisely by making an extra batch of these finger lickin' good chile rellenos and freezing them. That way they're at the ready when you're in a crunch for time but yearning for a homey, satisfying lunch.

**SERVES 4**
**PREP TIME:** 15 minutes
**COOK TIME:** 50 minutes

1 tablespoon olive oil

1 pound ground chicken

2 teaspoons chili powder

2 teaspoons ground cumin

¾ teaspoon ground coriander

¾ teaspoon garlic salt

½ teaspoon onion powder

½ teaspoon paprika

½ teaspoon dried oregano

½ teaspoon freshly ground black pepper

Cooking spray

4 fresh Anaheim chiles

8 ounces Pepper Jack cheese, cut into
   8 pieces

3 large eggs

1 cup heavy cream

1 teaspoon kosher salt

6 ounces shredded sharp cheddar cheese

1. In a large skillet, heat the oil over medium heat. Add the chicken, chili powder, cumin, coriander, garlic salt, onion powder, paprika, oregano, and pepper and cook, stirring frequently, and breaking the mixture up, until cooked through, about 5 minutes.

2. Preheat the oven to 350°F. Spray a 9 × 9-inch baking dish with cooking spray.

3. In a steamer set over a pan of simmering water, steam the chiles until softened, about 5 minutes. Halve the chiles lengthwise, arrange cut sides up in the prepared baking dish, and place a piece of cheese into each chile half.

4. In a small bowl, beat together the eggs, cream, and salt until well combined and pour the mixture over the chiles. Scatter the cooked chicken over the top and sprinkle the cheese over the chicken. Cover with foil and bake for 20 minutes. Uncover and bake until the custard is set, 15 to 20 minutes more. Serve hot.

# Chicken Cheese Quesadilla

To all the people out there who look at you with pity in their eyes thinking you now have to say goodbye to quesadillas, think again! Just whip up a batch of simple, easy, and delicious Chi-Keto-Friendly Tortillas and remember me when the burst of flavors hits your palate. Don't forget to add some Valentina hot sauce. It's all about enjoying what we eat so we want to keep coming back for more.

**SERVES 1**
**PREP TIME:** 10 minutes
**COOK TIME:** 10 minutes

3 ounces boneless, skinless chicken breast, cut into ½-inch chunks

1 teaspoon ground cumin

1 teaspoon dried oregano

½ teaspoon kosher salt

5 teaspoons avocado oil

½ small yellow onion, finely chopped (about ¼ cup)

½ small green bell pepper, finely chopped (about ¼ cup)

1 teaspoon chili powder

2 Chi-Keto-Friendly Tortillas (page 54)

⅓ cup shredded mozzarella cheese

1. In a medium bowl, toss the chicken with the cumin, oregano, and salt.

2. In a small skillet, heat 3 teaspoons of the oil over medium heat and sauté the onion, bell pepper, and chili powder for 3 minutes. Add the chicken and cook, stirring occasionally, until the chicken is cooked through, 3 to 4 minutes.

3. In another small skillet, heat the remaining 2 teaspoons oil over medium-low heat. Add one tortilla, then top with the chicken mixture and cheese. Place the other tortilla on top and cook until the cheese has melted, about 3 minutes. Cut in half to serve.

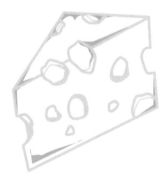

# Spicy Mozzarella Chicken Burger Ranch Salad

Here's another recipe that you can add to your Sunday meal prep for a time-saving meal when you're on the go during the week. Make the patties ahead of time, put the ones you will be using within the next day in the fridge, and freeze the rest to have them ready to cook in a pinch. These patties are so versatile; they're delicious in this salad, but you can also throw them on a grill and turn them into chicken burgers for your family and friends (wrapped in lettuce for you, of course). They're quick and easy and filling.

**SERVES 4**
**PREP TIME:** 20 minutes
**RESTING TIME FOR DRESSING:**
  30 minutes to overnight
**COOK TIME:** 15 minutes

1 pound ground chicken
½ cup finely chopped yellow onion
1 tablespoon garlic powder
1 teaspoon kosher salt
1 cup shredded mozzarella cheese
1 cup finely chopped baby spinach
½ cup finely chopped parsley
1 jalapeño, finely chopped (ribs and seeds removed for less heat, if desired)
2 tablespoons olive oil
1 cup chopped iceberg lettuce
½ avocado, pitted, peeled, and diced
1 Persian (mini) cucumber, diced
Ranch Dressing (page 101)

1. In a large bowl, combine the chicken, onion, garlic powder, salt, cheese, spinach, parsley, and jalapeño. Shape into eight 2½ × ½-inch patties.

2. In a large nonstick skillet, working in batches if necessary, heat the oil over medium heat, add the patties, and cook until cooked through, about 4 minutes per side.

3. In a medium bowl, combine the lettuce, avocado, and cucumber. Add ¼ cup of the dressing and toss to coat. Divide among four plates, top each with two patties and serve.

## Ranch Dressing
**MAKES 1½ CUPS**

½ cup mayonnaise
½ cup heavy cream
½ cup sour cream
1 teaspoon lemon juice
½ teaspoon dried chives
1 teaspoon chopped fresh parsley or
   ½ teaspoon dried
1 teaspoon chopped fresh dill or
   ½ teaspoon dried dill weed
½ teaspoon garlic powder
¼ teaspoon onion powder
⅛ teaspoon kosher salt
⅛ teaspoon freshly ground black pepper

In a large bowl, whisk together all the ingredients. Cover and refrigerate for at least 30 minutes. It tastes even better if you refrigerate it overnight.

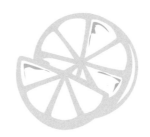

# Stuffed Zucchini Boats

Bubbling cheese, salsa, juicy ground turkey . . . just thinking about it makes my mouth water. Because this recipe is a little bit more tedious to make, it is another meal-prep gem. If you're going to cook something like this, make the most of your time by doubling the recipe and freezing the leftovers. Want to change it up next time you have these zucchini boats? Add some Parmesan cheese and crushed chili peppers to turn it into a lasagna-pizza hybrid and satisfy two cravings in one!

**SERVES 6**
**PREP TIME:** 15 minutes
**COOK TIME:** 40 minutes

Cooking spray
3 medium zucchini (6 to 7 ounces each), halved lengthwise and seeds removed
1 tablespoon olive oil
2 cloves garlic, finely chopped
1½ pounds (85% lean) ground turkey
1 teaspoon ground cumin
1 teaspoon smoked paprika
¾ teaspoon kosher salt
½ teaspoon chili powder
½ teaspoon onion powder
¼ teaspoon garlic powder
¼ teaspoon dried oregano
1 cup salsa
1½ cups shredded Mexican cheese blend
Sour cream, for garnish
Chopped cilantro, for garnish

1. Preheat the oven to 400°F. Spray a 9 × 13-inch baking dish with cooking spray.
2. Place the zucchini cut side down in the prepared baking dish and bake until crisp-tender, about 10 minutes.
3. In a large skillet, heat the oil over medium heat. Add the garlic and cook 1 minute. Add the turkey and cook 1 to 2 minutes, stirring to break up any lumps. Add the cumin, paprika, salt, chili powder, onion powder, garlic powder, and oregano and stir to combine. Add the salsa and 1 cup of the cheese and cook until the cheese has melted, about 1 minute.
4. Turn the zucchini cut side up, fill each with the turkey mixture, cover with foil, and bake for 20 minutes or until the zucchini are tender. Uncover, top with the remaining cheese, and bake 1 minute longer or until the cheese has melted. Top each zucchini boat with sour cream and cilantro.

# Tuna Bacon Salad

Many mornings I wake up and hit the ground running. I may not even leave my house, but I'm on calls, texting, and preparing for future projects, and then I blink and it's lunchtime. It can hit you by surprise and you won't have time to make anything elaborate on those crazy busy days. With this salad, all you need is 10 minutes and you're good to go. That's why it's the one you can turn to when you need to put something together in a flash that will keep you nourished and satisfied, but also keep your energy high so you can boss-bee the hell out of the rest of the day!

**SERVES 2**

**PREP TIME:** 10 minutes

3 tablespoons mayonnaise

2 tablespoons lemon juice

1 teaspoon Dijon mustard

½ teaspoon kosher salt

2 (5-ounce) cans tuna, packed in olive oil

2 slices bacon, cooked and crumbled

2 stalks celery, finely chopped

3 scallions, thinly sliced

1 tablespoon chopped fresh dill

1½ cups arugula

1. In a medium bowl, combine the mayonnaise, lemon juice, Dijon, and salt. Add the tuna, bacon, celery, scallions, and dill and mix together.
2. Divide the arugula between two bowls, top with the tuna, and serve.
3. You can also turn it into a sandwich with keto zero-net-carb bread you can find in the grocery store.

# Steak Fajita Rolls

I love sandwiches and I love fajitas, so this is like a match made in heaven. The flavor combination of steak, bell pepper, and onion will make you forget you ever needed tortillas with this dish before. To top it off, it's another quick-and-easy lunch to have when you're navigating one of those days where you can't skip a beat. To make it even easier, marinate ahead of time so it's ready to go.

SERVES 4 (2 to 3 rolls per serving)
PREP TIME: 15 minutes
MARINATING TIME: 30 minutes to
  overnight
COOK TIME: 10 minutes

⅓ cup olive oil

3 tablespoons Worcestershire sauce

2 tablespoons fresh lime juice

2 cloves garlic, finely chopped

1 tablespoon ground cumin

1 tablespoon chili powder

1 teaspoon kosher salt

½ teaspoon freshly ground black pepper

½ teaspoon red pepper flakes

1-pound sirloin steak, sliced extra thin
  and pounded flat

2 yellow bell peppers, thinly sliced

½ medium red onion, thinly sliced

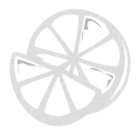

1. In a medium bowl, whisk together the oil, Worcestershire, lime juice, garlic, cumin, chili powder, salt, black pepper, and red pepper flakes.

2. Divide the mixture between two large zip-top resealable bags. Place the meat in one and the bell peppers and onion in another. Shake the bags to coat the meat and the bell peppers and onion with the marinade. Refrigerate at least 30 minutes, or up to overnight (the longer the marinating time, the more flavorful the meat).

3. Preheat the oven to 375°F. Line a rimmed sheet pan with parchment paper.

4. Lift the meat from the marinade and lay the slices on the prepared sheet pan. Remove the bell peppers and onion from the marinade and divide them among the slices of meat, arranging them crosswise. Roll the meat up and secure with toothpicks.

5. Bake until the meat is cooked to your liking, about 10 minutes for medium. If you have extra veggies, cook them on the sheet pan along with the meat. Remove the toothpicks and serve.

# Bacon Guacamole Chicken Bomb

Another delicious bomb, this time for lunch! Guacamole stuffed into chicken and then wrapped with bacon? I am all in! Bonus: if you have guacamole to spare, use it as a topping for any of the salads or tacos in this book, or dip some bell pepper strips into it and have it as a snack, or add a dollop to an omelet. You can honestly put guacamole on anything, so I suggest you make an extra batch and have it at the ready.

**SERVES 4**
**PREP TIME:** 15 minutes
**COOK TIME:** 25 minutes

4 boneless, skinless chicken breasts
 (6 ounces each)
1 teaspoon kosher salt
½ teaspoon freshly ground black pepper
Guacamole (page 106)
8 slices bacon (not thick cut)
1 tablespoon olive oil

1. Preheat the oven to 425°F.
2. Place the chicken on a cutting board and, with a chef's knife, cut into the thickest part, making a slit about 3 inches long. Wiggle the knife to cut about three-quarters of the way into the chicken without cutting through to the other side. Season the chicken with the salt and pepper.
3. Spoon the guacamole into a pastry bag without a tip and pipe about 2 tablespoons of the guacamole into the pocket of each chicken breast. Wrap each chicken breast tightly with 2 slices of bacon and secure with toothpicks.
4. In a large ovenproof skillet, heat the oil over medium heat. Place the chicken in the skillet and sear each breast on one side, 3 to 4 minutes. Turn the chicken breasts over, transfer to the oven, and bake until the bacon is crisp and the chicken is cooked through, about 20 minutes.

## Guacamole

2 avocados, halved, pitted, and peeled
⅓ cup coarsely chopped tomato
¼ cup finely chopped white onion
2 tablespoons chopped fresh cilantro
4 teaspoons fresh lime juice
½ teaspoon kosher salt

In a large bowl, with a potato masher, mash the avocados. Stir in the tomato, onion, cilantro, lime juice, and salt.

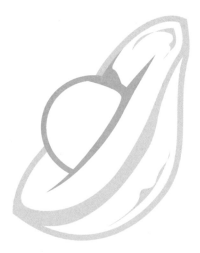

# Shrimp Stir-Fry

I think I was Asian in another life. If you put me on a deserted island and said I had only one type of food to choose from, I'd say anything Asian, hands down. I've always been intrigued by Asian culture and cuisine, and I could easily have Asian food—anything and everything from Vietnamese to Thai to Korean—every day for the rest of my life. Thankfully, my husband, Lorenzo, loves it too, so much so that sometimes we have it twice a day! I was actually a pescatarian for a long time, and my go-to meals then were filled with fish and shrimp, so this stir-fry speaks to my heart in more ways than one.

**SERVES 1**
**PREP TIME:** 15 minutes
**COOK TIME:** 10 minutes

2½ tablespoons liquid aminos

1 tablespoon toasted sesame oil

1 teaspoon sriracha (more if you'd like it spicier)

1½ teaspoons finely chopped garlic

1½ teaspoons finely chopped fresh ginger

¼ teaspoon red pepper flakes

2 tablespoons coconut oil

1 cup broccoli florets

½ cup thinly sliced carrots

½ pound large shrimp (about 9), peeled and deveined

2 tablespoons hemp seeds

1 teaspoon sesame seeds

1. In a small bowl, mix together the liquid aminos, sesame oil, sriracha, garlic, ginger, and red pepper flakes.

2. In a large skillet, heat the coconut oil over medium heat. Add the broccoli and carrots and cook until the carrots are crisp-tender, about 2 minutes. Add the shrimp and sauce and cook, stirring frequently, until the shrimp are just cooked through, 3 to 4 minutes.

3. Add the hemp seeds and sesame seeds and toss to combine.

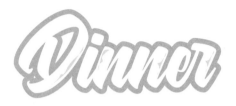

# Dinner

*The kitchen is the heart of my home. It's a place where I can come together with myself and with my family, give thanks for the ups, the downs, and the lessons learned throughout the day, and simply unwind. Dinner is a perfect time to slow down and cook up some delicious food for yourself and your loved ones, and to reflect on and celebrate the close of yet another day on earth. My favorites for the evening are the mouthwatering Carne a la Tampiqueña with Roasted Zucchini (page 129) and my all-time favorite, Chicken Taquitos (page 137), which reminds me of my mom.*

## Chingona Tip

After a long day, sometimes all we want is to unwind with a glass of wine with dinner. That's okay. Just make sure you stick to only one 5-ounce serving and pick the drier varieties, such as a Pinot Noir or a Sauvignon Blanc, or even a flute of champagne. If you're a tequila lover like me, that's what the Happy Hour section (pages 141 to 146) is for, baby . . . ¡salud!

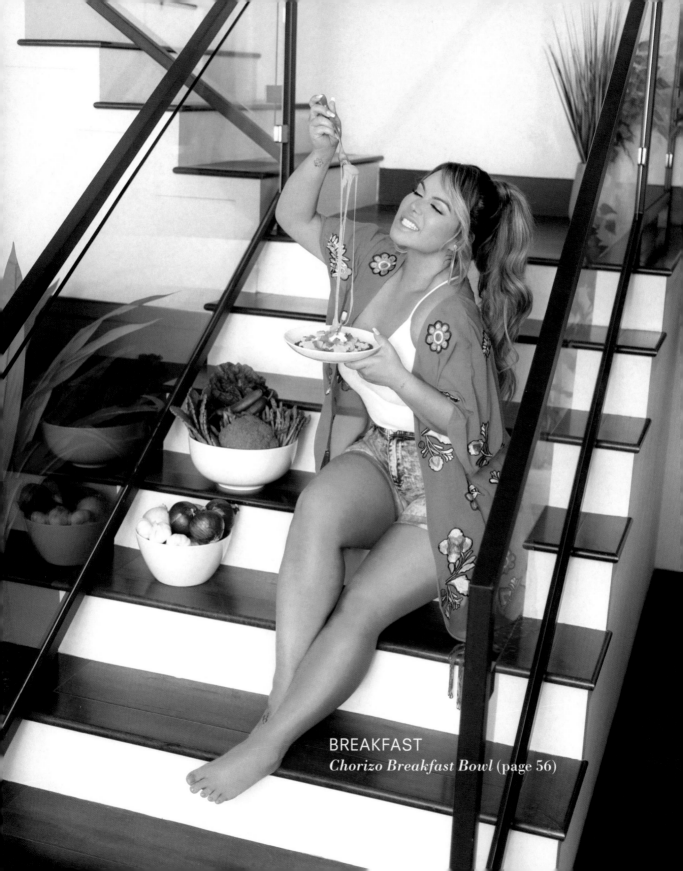

BREAKFAST
*Chorizo Breakfast Bowl* (page 56)

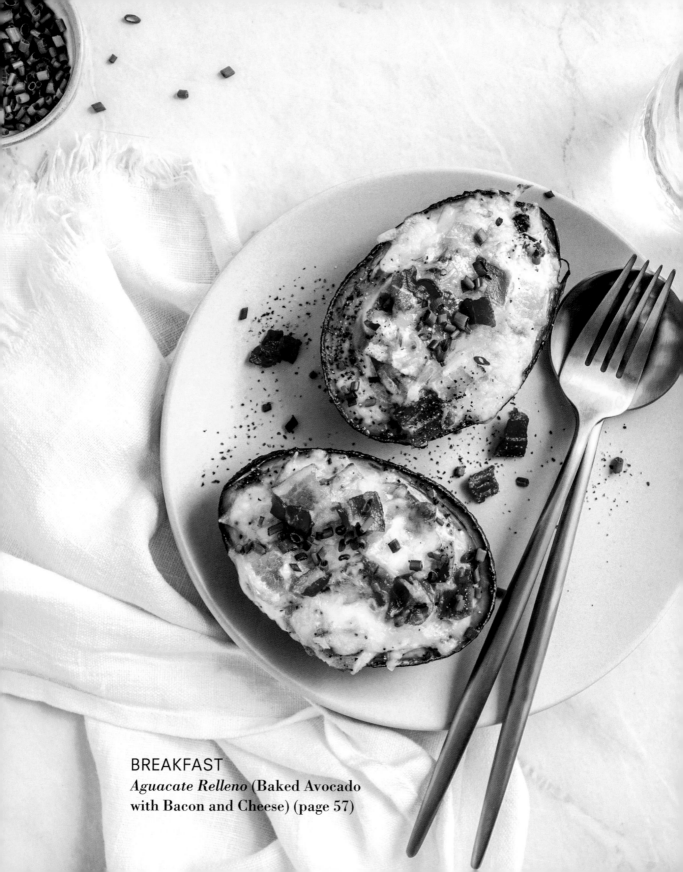

BREAKFAST
*Aguacate Relleno* (Baked Avocado
with Bacon and Cheese) (page 57)

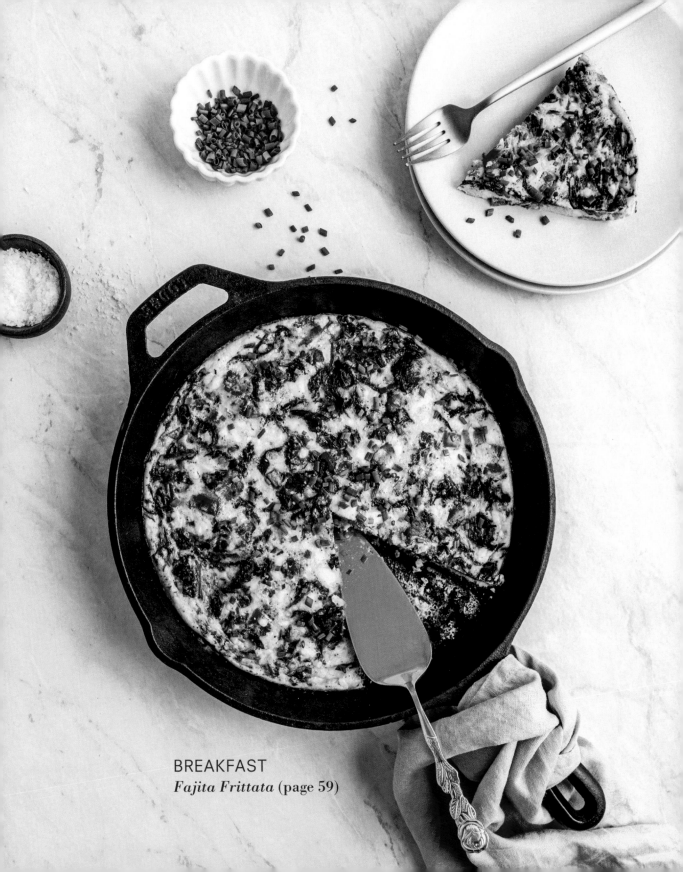

BREAKFAST
*Fajita Frittata* (page 59)

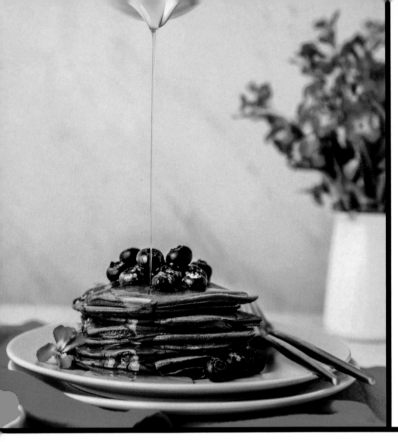

BREAKFAST
*Chocolate Blueberry Pancakes*
(page 62)

BREAKFAST
*Pumpkin Spice Coffee Smoothie*
(page 74)

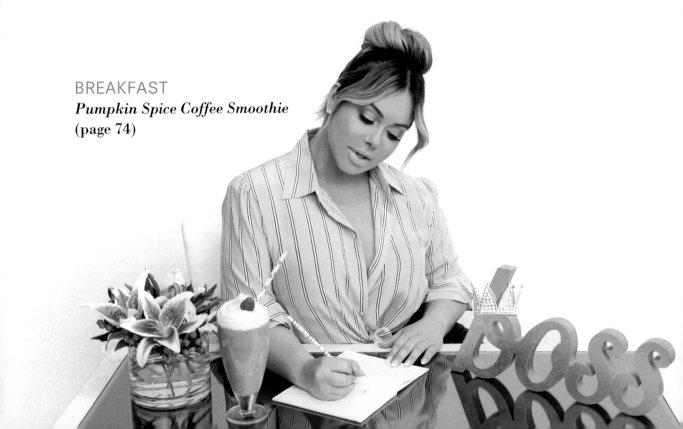

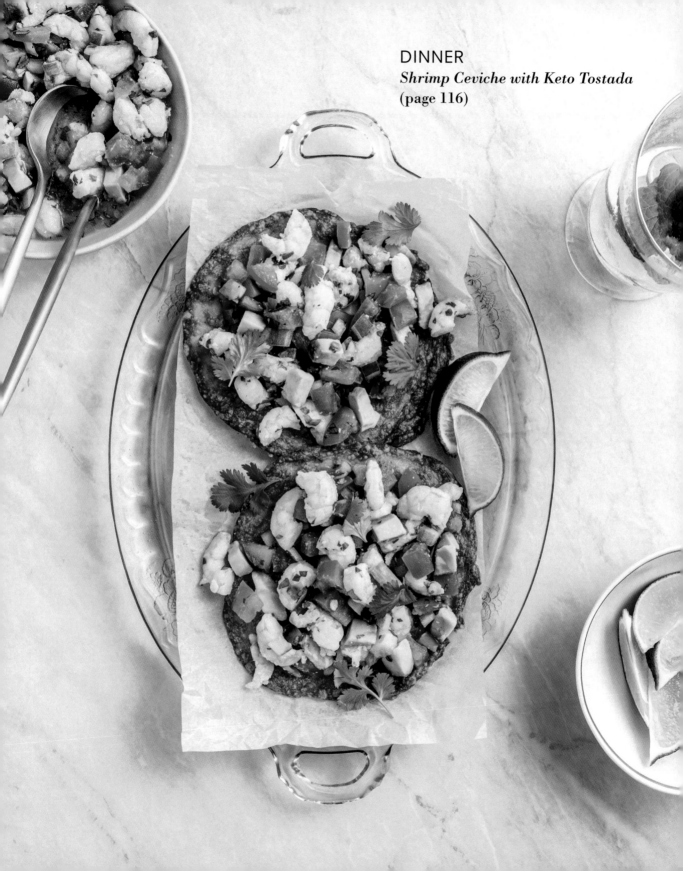

DINNER
*Shrimp Ceviche with Keto Tostada*
(page 116)

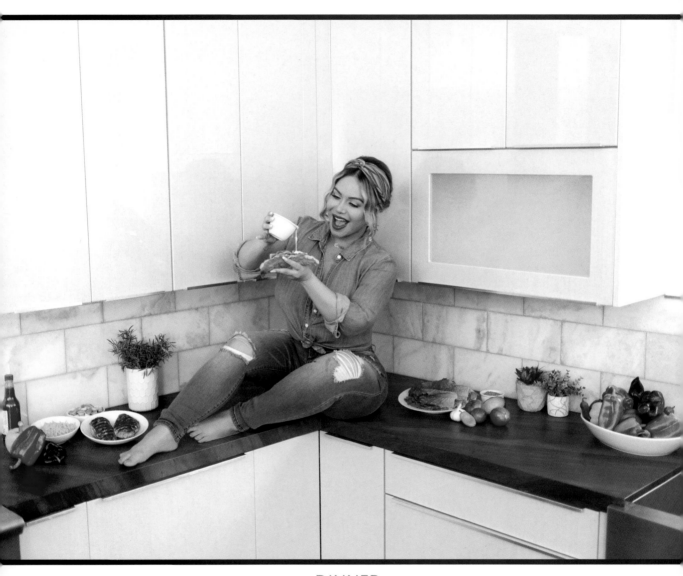

DINNER
*Chi-Keto Tacos* (Lettuce-Wrapped Chicken Tacos
with Cilantro Crema) (page 111)

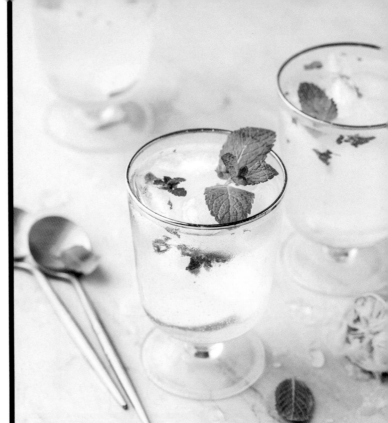

HAPPY HOUR
*Ay Mojito, Qué Rico*
**(page 143)**

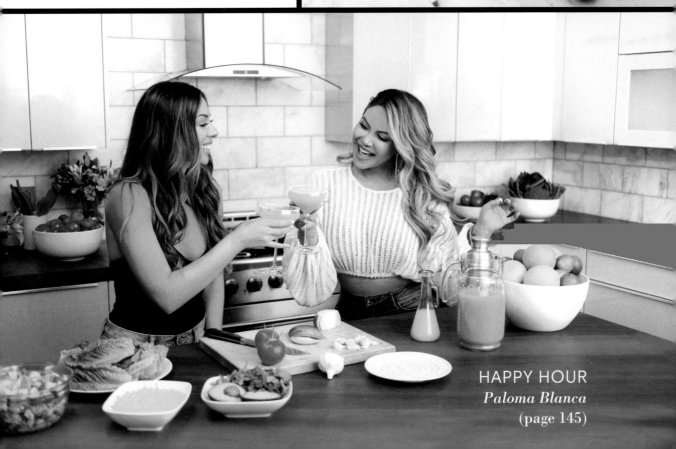

HAPPY HOUR
*Paloma Blanca*
**(page 145)**

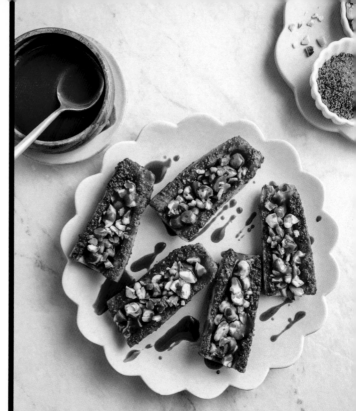

SNACKS
*Pepinos Locos*
(page 150)

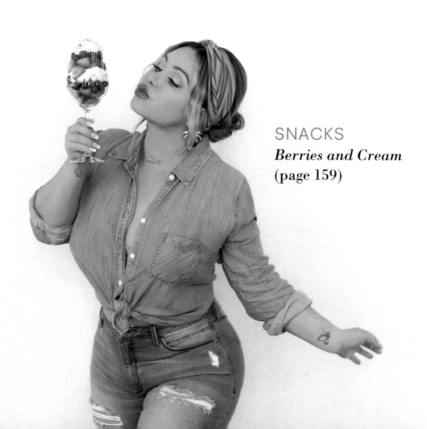

SNACKS
*Berries and Cream*
(page 159)

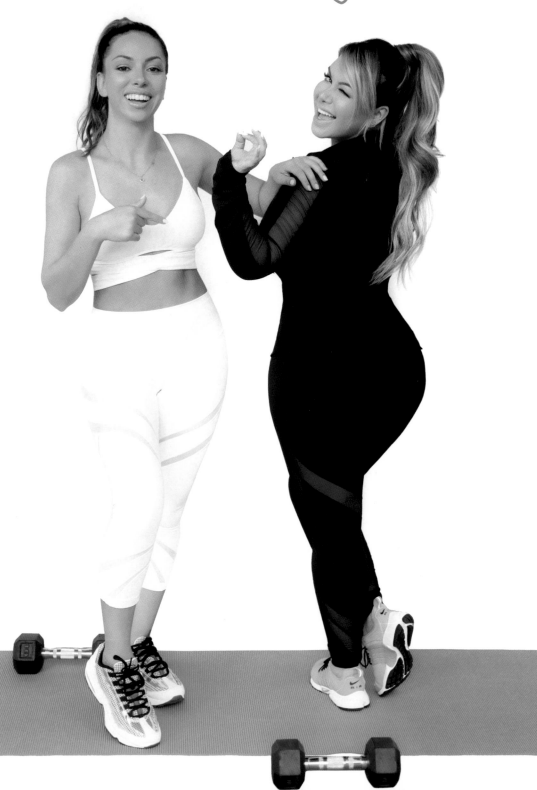

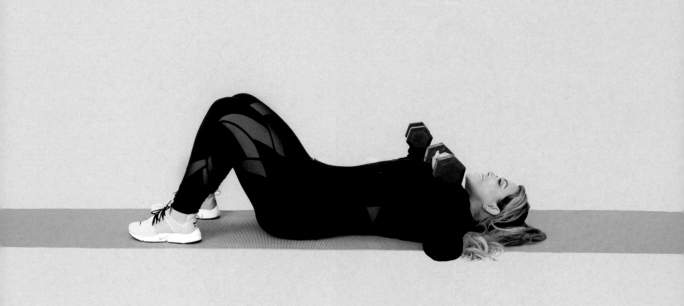

*Variation for Week 3, Workout 1: Glute Bridges to Chest Presses* (page 163)

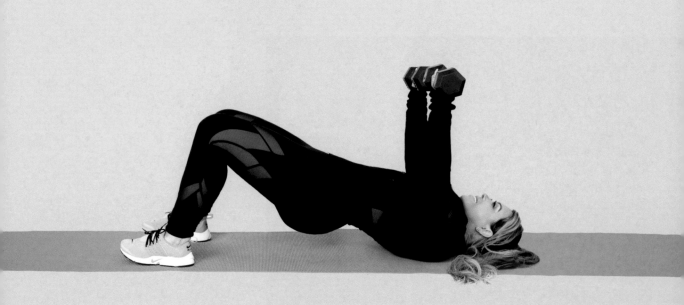

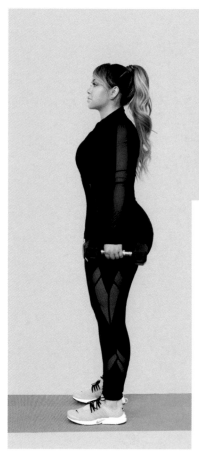

*Variation for Week 2, Workout 1:*
*Dumbbell Squats (page 165)*

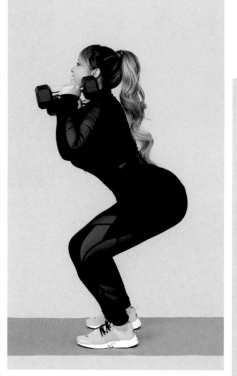

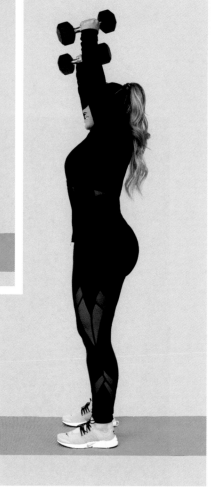

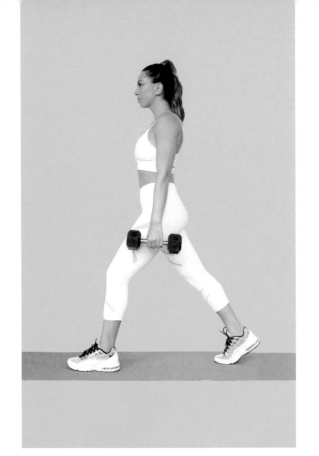

*Variation for Week 3, Workout 2:*
*Stagnant Lunges to Bicep Curls* (page 166)

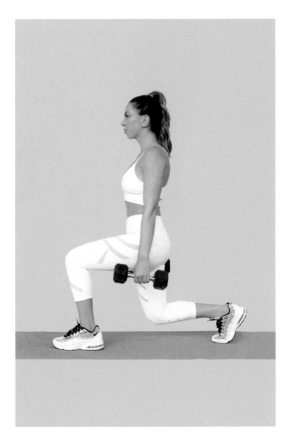

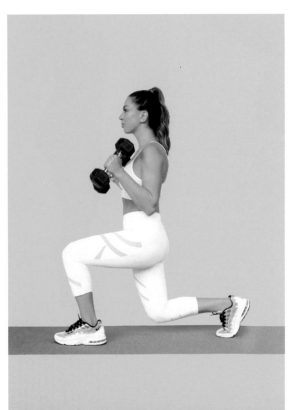

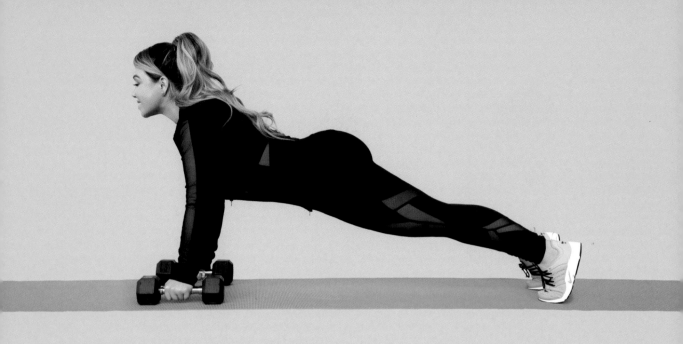

*Variation for Week 3, Workout 2: Plank Rows* (page 167)

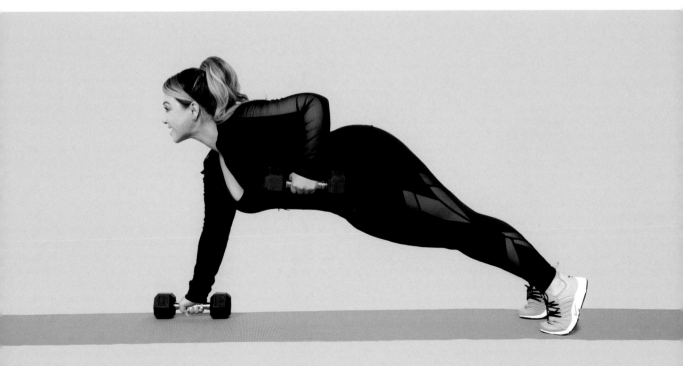

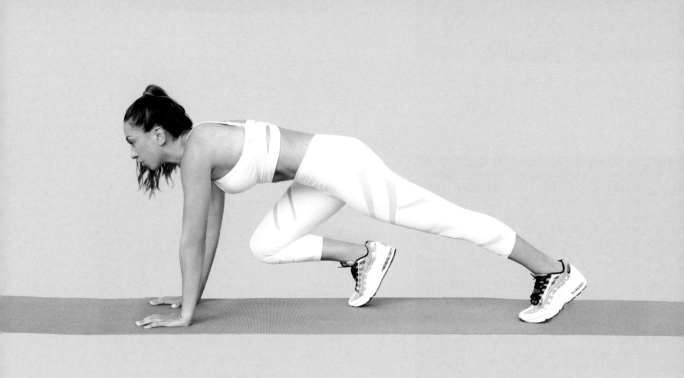

*Essential Exercise 9: Mountain Climbers* (page 168)

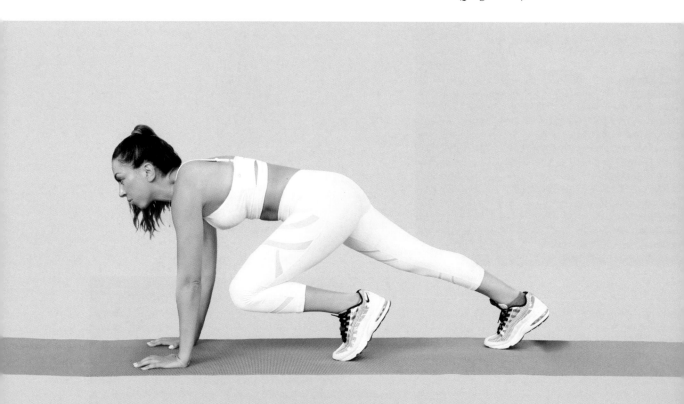

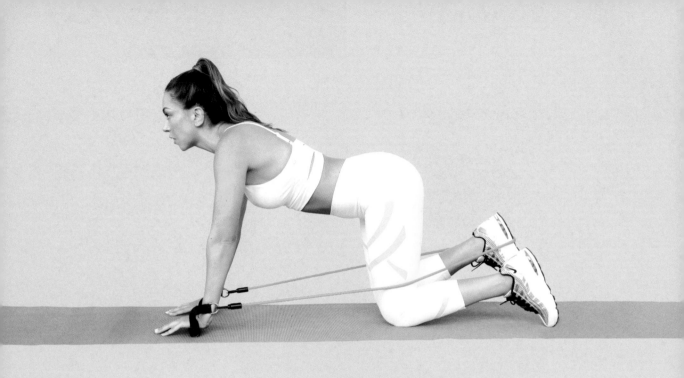

*Variation for Weeks 2 and 3, Workout 3: Banded Glute Kickbacks* (page 169)

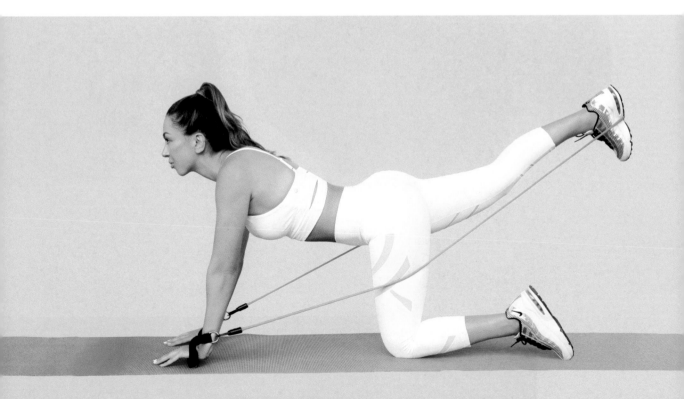

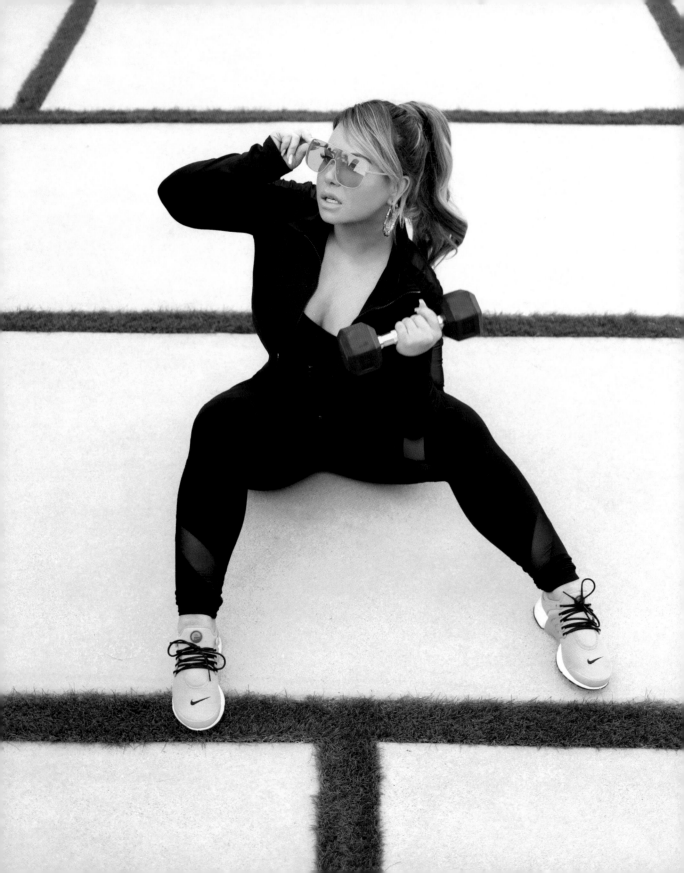

# *Chi-Keto Tacos* (Lettuce-Wrapped Chicken Tacos with Cilantro Crema)

Did I mention I love tacos? I can't get enough of them, and now I no longer have to miss out on Taco Tuesdays with this super-easy and simple dinner. The lettuce takes the place of the tortilla and holds the juicy chicken and tomato, onion, avocado, cheese, and cilantro crema. Um, did someone say diet? No, girl, this is a lifestyle, and life is made to be filled with flavor and joy like these tacos.

**SERVES 4**
**PREP TIME:** 15 minutes
**MARINATING TIME:** 20 minutes to
24 hours
**COOK TIME:** 10 minutes

1 pound boneless, skinless chicken breasts

2 tablespoons taco seasoning

2 cloves garlic, finely chopped

1 tablespoon avocado oil, plus more for the grill

8 romaine lettuce leaves

1 avocado, halved, pitted, peeled, and diced

½ medium yellow onion, diced

1 medium tomato, diced

2 tablespoons shredded cheese of choice

Cilantro Crema (page 112)

Hot sauce of choice, if desired

1. In a large bowl, toss the chicken with the taco seasoning, garlic, and oil. Cover and refrigerate for 20 minutes, or up to 24 hours.

2. Lightly oil the grill grates of a grill and heat to medium or heat a skillet with 1 to 2 tablespoons of oil over medium heat. Cut the chicken into strips. Grill the chicken until cooked through, about 5 minutes per side. Transfer to a cutting board and thinly slice.

3. Arrange the lettuce on a platter and top with the chicken, avocado, onion, tomato, and cheese. Drizzle with the crema and serve.

## Cilantro Crema

½ cup Mexican crema
2 tablespoons olive oil
1 tablespoon fresh lime juice
½ cup packed cilantro leaves
1 jalapeño (ribs and seeds removed for
  less heat, if desired)
1 clove garlic
¼ teaspoon kosher salt

In a blender, puree all the ingredients until smooth.

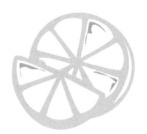

# *Fajitas a la Flor* (Chicken Fajitas with Mexican Cauliflower Rice)

One of my favorite Mexican dishes is fajitas with rice. But rice doesn't sit well in my stomach, so finding an alternative was a top priority. At first, I was a little skeptical about cauliflower rice. I used to choose broccoli over cauliflower any day—especially since eating steamed whole cauliflower florets usually made me pretty gassy—until I tried cauliflower rice. It's super light, and I love that I can transform it into an *arroz rojo*—most Mexican homes have a side of red rice ready to accompany anything else on the stove— and still have something that has a similar texture to rice without the uncomfortable side effects.

**SERVES 4**
**PREP TIME:** 15 minutes
**COOK TIME:** 25 minutes

*For the chicken*
2 teaspoons chili powder
2 teaspoons smoked paprika
1 teaspoon ground cumin
1 teaspoon garlic powder
2 tablespoons plus 1 teaspoon avocado oil
5 teaspoons fresh lime juice, plus more for serving
1 pound boneless, skinless chicken breasts (6 ounces each), sliced ½ inch thick crosswise
2 tablespoons grass-fed butter
1 medium yellow onion, halved and thinly sliced
1 medium red bell pepper, thinly sliced
1 medium green bell pepper, thinly sliced
1 medium yellow bell pepper, thinly sliced
Kosher salt to taste

*For the cauliflower rice*
⅔ cup chicken broth
1 cup canned or fresh diced tomatoes
¼ medium yellow onion, diced
1 jalapeño with seeds, finely chopped
3 tablespoons taco seasoning
12 ounces fresh or frozen and thawed cauliflower rice
2 cups shredded sharp cheddar cheese
½ cup sour cream
½ avocado, pitted, peeled, and sliced

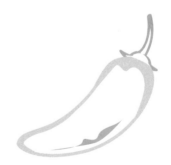

1. *For the chicken*: In a small bowl, combine the chili powder, paprika, cumin, and garlic powder.

2. In a large bowl, whisk together 2 tablespoons of the oil, the lime juice, and 5 teaspoons of the spice mixture. Add the chicken and toss to coat.

3. In a large nonstick skillet, heat the butter and the remaining 1 teaspoon oil over medium heat. Add the onion and cook, stirring occasionally, until crisp-tender, about 3 minutes. Add the bell peppers and the remaining spice mixture and cook, stirring occasionally, until crisp-tender, about 5 minutes. Transfer to a bowl.

4. Add the chicken to the skillet, season with salt, and sauté until cooked through, 3 to 4 minutes.

5. *For the cauliflower rice*: In another large skillet, bring the broth, tomatoes, onion, jalapeño, and taco seasoning to a simmer over medium heat. Stir in the cauliflower rice, reduce the heat to medium-low, cover, and cook until the cauliflower is tender, 7 to 10 minutes.

6. Add 1½ cups of the cheese, replace the cover, and let stand until the cheese has melted, about 1 minute. Divide the cauliflower rice among four plates, top with the chicken mixture, sour cream, the remaining ½ cup of cheese, the avocado, and a drizzle of lime juice and serve.

# *Nacho-Bitch* (Cauliflower Chorizo over Chicharrón Nachos)

Nachos are the bomb. They're super easy to make and satisfying and usually the ultimate junk food. I used to have them as an appetizer followed by my main dish. Thankfully, my Chi-Keto lifestyle has taught me how to eat less while still remaining comfortably fulfilled; that's why I now consider this a main dish, not a snack. Nacho-Bitch not only helps me satisfy this particular craving, it also makes me feel like I can still have fun with my food, and that's priceless.

**SERVES 2**
**PREP TIME:** 10 minutes
**COOK TIME:** 35 minutes

1 large head cauliflower, (about 2½ pounds) cored and coarsely chopped
3 tablespoons olive oil
¾ teaspoon ground cumin
¾ teaspoon paprika
¾ teaspoon kosher salt
½ teaspoon chili powder
½ teaspoon garlic powder
1 cup shredded Colby Jack cheese
2 teaspoons ghee
2 fresh sweet or hot chorizos, casings removed

*Toppings*
Salsa
Guacamole (page 106)
Sliced pickled jalapeños
Sour cream

1. Preheat the oven to 450°F.
2. In a baking pan, toss the cauliflower with the oil, cumin, paprika, salt, chili powder, and garlic powder until nicely coated. Bake, tossing occasionally, until the cauliflower is tender, about 25 minutes. Scatter the cheese over the cauliflower, return the pan to the oven, and bake until the cheese has melted, about 5 minutes more.
3. Meanwhile, in a small skillet, heat the ghee over medium heat. Add the chorizos, crumbling them with a fork and cook, stirring occasionally, until cooked through, about 3 minutes.
4. Scatter the chorizos over the cauliflower and serve with your choice of toppings.

# Shrimp Ceviche with Keto Tostada

Walking back from the beach with the sand clinging to my toes, my skin hot from soaking in the rays, one of my favorite go-to lunches is a refreshing ceviche. This reminds me of a summer beach day but with a Mexican kick, because the shrimp is all limey and juicy . . . and the crunch of those mozzarella tostadas is everything.

**SERVES 2**
**PREP TIME:** 10 minutes
**MARINATING TIME:** 15 minutes
**COOK TIME:** 10 minutes

½ cup fresh orange juice (from 2 to 3 juice oranges)

6 tablespoons fresh lime juice (from 2 to 3 limes)

6 tablespoons fresh lemon juice (from 2 lemons)

1 pound large cooked shrimp (about 18), cut into thirds crosswise

3 Roma (plum) tomatoes, diced

½ cup chopped fresh cilantro

¼ cup finely chopped red onion

2 serrano peppers, seeded and finely chopped (about 4 teaspoons)

1 avocado, halved, pitted, peeled, and diced

Kosher salt to taste

Mozzarella Tostadas (page 80)

1. In a small bowl, whisk together the orange, lime, and lemon juices. Transfer half to a large bowl, add the shrimp, and toss to coat. Let stand for 15 minutes.

2. Add the tomatoes, cilantro, onion, and serranos; toss to combine. Add the remaining juice mixture and the avocado, season with salt, and toss gently to combine. Serve with mozzarella tostadas.

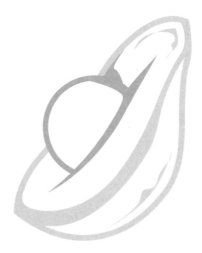

## *Pollo a la Plancha* (Grilled Chicken with Lemon Arugula Parmesan Salad)

Remember that bland AF chicken I talked about hating in the introduction? Well, as you can imagine, I wasn't going to make you suffer through that here. This is a grilled chicken with a kick. Something you'll actually look forward to eating. And the tanginess of the lemon arugula Parmesan salad combo is pure healthy deliciousness.

**SERVES 4**
**PREP TIME:** 10 minutes
**MARINATING TIME:** 3 hours to overnight
**COOK TIME:** 6 minutes

4 boneless, skinless chicken breasts (6 ounces each)
1½ cups chopped yellow onion
4 scallions, thinly sliced
7 cloves garlic, crushed and peeled
¾ cup dark beer
2¾ teaspoons ground cumin
½ teaspoon kosher salt
¼ teaspoon freshly ground black pepper
¼ teaspoon ground achiote
Olive oil
1 tablespoon fresh lemon juice
2 cups arugula
2 tablespoons shaved Parmesan cheese

1. With a meat mallet or the bottom of a heavy skillet, pound the chicken breasts to an even ½-inch thickness.

2. In a blender, puree the onion, scallions, garlic, beer, cumin, salt, pepper, and achiote until smooth. Transfer to a shallow bowl, add the chicken, and toss to coat. Cover and refrigerate at least 3 hours, or up to overnight.

3. Lightly oil the grill grates of a grill and heat to medium. Grill the chicken, turning it once, until cooked through, 2 to 3 minutes per side. (If you don't have a grill, use a grill pan or a skillet.)

4. In a medium bowl, whisk together 2 teaspoons olive oil and the lemon juice. Add the arugula, toss to coat, and top with the Parmesan. Serve alongside the chicken.

# Roasted Salmon with Lime Cream Sauce and Asparagus

As much as I love seafood, I'll be honest, salmon is not my first choice. However, I know how amazing it is health-wise and that it's also incredibly filling, so it's important to include it in our day-to-day living and in this book, especially for all you salmon lovers out there! Salmon is the perfect keto-friendly food. It's a protein that's filled with wonderful good-for-you fat. Add the asparagus and you've got yourself a perfectly balanced meal that will keep you satiated and happy.

**SERVES 4**
**PREP TIME:** 15 minutes
**MARINATING TIME:** 10 minutes
**COOK TIME:** 15 minutes

½ cup Mexican crema

½ teaspoon finely grated lime zest

4 teaspoons fresh lime juice

¼ cup finely chopped cilantro

2 scallions, thinly sliced (about ¼ cup)

Kosher salt

1 teaspoon chili powder

1 clove garlic, minced

2 tablespoons olive oil

4 skin-on salmon fillets (5 ounces each)

1 bunch asparagus (about 1 pound), tough ends trimmed and cut into 1-inch pieces

1 teaspoon smoked paprika

½ teaspoon garlic powder

2 tablespoons red wine vinegar

1. In a small bowl, whisk together the crema, lime zest, 2 teaspoons of the lime juice, the cilantro, scallions, and ½ teaspoon salt.

2. In another small bowl, combine the chili powder, garlic, 1 tablespoon of the oil, the remaining 2 teaspoons lime juice, and ¼ teaspoon salt. Spoon the mixture over the skinless sides of the salmon and let stand for 10 minutes.

3. Preheat the oven to 450°F.

4. Place the salmon skin side down on a small rimmed sheet pan or in an oven-proof skillet and cook to desired degree of doneness, about 10 minutes for medium (timing will vary depending on the thickness of the fish). Transfer to a serving platter.

5. Meanwhile, in a large skillet, heat the remaining 1 tablespoon oil over medium-high heat. Add the asparagus and 2 tablespoons water and cook, stirring frequently, until almost tender, about 4 minutes (timing will vary depending on the thickness of the asparagus).

6. Add the paprika, garlic powder, and ¼ teaspoon salt and cook until crisp-tender, about 1 minute.

7. Add the vinegar, toss to coat, and transfer the asparagus to the platter with the salmon. Spoon the sauce over the salmon and serve.

# Fried Chicken with Mashed Garlic Cauliflower

When I am about to get my period or on it, I crave fried food like there's no tomorrow. That's why I love this alternative. It totally gives me the fried-food comfort I need without the extra calories or bloat—and you know we don't need any more bloating during that time of the month! I also turn to this recipe on game day, so that while everyone else is scarfing down pizza and fried chicken I don't feel left out.

**SERVES 2 (2 pieces of chicken and 1 cup of mashed garlic cauliflower per serving)**

**PREP TIME:** 25 minutes
**COOK TIME:** 40 minutes

Cooking spray

4 ounces chicharrón

1½ teaspoons dried thyme

1⅛ teaspoons freshly ground black pepper to taste

1 teaspoon kosher salt

1 teaspoon dried oregano

1 teaspoon smoked paprika

½ teaspoon plus 1 tablespoon garlic powder

1 large egg

¼ cup mayonnaise

3 tablespoons Dijon mustard

4 skinless chicken legs (10 ounces each), drumsticks and thighs separated

1 clove garlic, smashed

1 head cauliflower, cut into small florets

½ cup half-and-half

½ cup shredded cheddar cheese

1 tablespoon cream cheese

1 tablespoon grass-fed butter

Chives for topping, if desired

1. Preheat the oven to 400°F. Set a wire rack inside a large baking pan. Spray the rack with cooking spray.

2. In a food processor, pulse the chicharrón along with the thyme, 1 teaspoon of the pepper, ½ teaspoon of the salt, the oregano, smoked paprika, and ½ teaspoon of the garlic powder. Transfer to a large plate.

3. In a large bowl, lightly beat the egg with the mayonnaise and Dijon.

4. Dip each piece of chicken first into the egg-mayo mixture, then into the chicharrón mixture, patting to coat completely. Place the chicken on the wire rack and bake until cooked through, about 40 minutes.

5. Meanwhile, in a large skillet, bring ½ cup water, the garlic, and the remaining ½ teaspoon salt and ⅛ teaspoon pepper to a boil. Add the cauliflower, cover, and cook over medium heat until very tender, about 15 minutes. Drain any remaining water.

6. Add the half-and-half, cheddar, cream cheese, butter, and the remaining 1 tablespoon garlic powder to the pan,

cover, and cook over medium-low heat
until the cheese has melted, about
2 minutes. With a potato masher, mash
the cauliflower to your desired consistency. Add chives, if desired and serve.

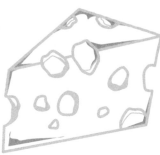

# Creamy Chicken Tomato Noodles

I love everything about Italian food . . . especially pasta! It's my comfort food. I started eating it with my first boyfriend when I was about nineteen years old. He was really into pasta and introduced me to lasagna and bowtie noodles. It was so important to us; our place, our thing, was going to Olive Garden. Even though I know it isn't good for me, I could still eat it every single day, which is why having a healthy alternative is sooo important to me. And when I am craving it hard, I simply treat myself with the real thing on my indulgence day.

**SERVES 1**
**PREP TIME:** 10 minutes
**COOK TIME:** 12 minutes

1 tablespoon grass-fed butter

1 chicken breast (6 ounces), cut into ½-inch chunks

1 tablespoon avocado oil

2 cloves garlic, crushed through a garlic press or finely chopped

8 ounces store-bought zoodles or 2 zucchini spiralized

4 ounces cream cheese, softened and cut into small chunks

2 tablespoons Mexican crema

½ cup sun-dried tomatoes packed in oil, coarsely chopped

¼ teaspoon dried oregano

¾ teaspoon kosher salt

¼ teaspoon freshly ground black pepper

2 tablespoons grated Parmesan cheese

2 tablespoons chopped fresh basil

1. In a large nonstick skillet, heat the butter over medium heat and sauté the chicken until just cooked through, about 4 minutes. With a slotted spoon, remove the chicken to a bowl.

2. Add the oil to the skillet and cook the garlic and zoodles, stirring frequently, until the zoodles are tender, about 3 minutes.

3. Stir in the cream cheese and crema and cook, stirring frequently, until the cream cheese has melted, about 2 minutes.

4. Add the chicken, sun-dried tomatoes, oregano, salt, and pepper and cook until heated through, about 3 minutes. Transfer to a plate or shallow bowl and top with the Parmesan and basil.

# Chicken Sausage Vegetable Skillet

When I'm craving breakfast for dinner, this is what I turn to. The sausage combined with the low-carb veggies and melted cheese are to die for. It's easy to make, nutritious, and filling. Switch it up and make it for breakfast one day too!

**SERVES 2**
**PREP TIME:** 10 minutes
**COOK TIME:** 20 minutes

2 tablespoons garlic ghee
2 fresh chicken sausage links (about 2¾ ounces each)
½ small red onion, cut into ½-inch chunks
1 clove garlic, finely chopped
1 small zucchini (4 ounces), halved lengthwise and thinly sliced
½ small red bell pepper, cut into ½-inch chunks
6 cremini mushrooms, sliced
½ teaspoon Italian seasoning
½ teaspoon red pepper flakes
Sea salt and freshly ground black pepper to taste
2 tablespoons grated Parmesan cheese

1. In a large skillet, heat the ghee over medium heat. Add the chicken sausage and cook until cooked through, about 7 minutes. Remove to a cutting board and when cool enough to handle, thinly slice.

2. Add the onion and garlic to the skillet and sauté until crisp-tender, about 7 minutes.

3. Add the sausage, zucchini, bell pepper, mushrooms, Italian seasoning, red pepper flakes, salt, and black pepper and cook until the vegetables are cooked through, about 5 minutes. Divide between 2 plates, sprinkle the cheese over and serve.

# Chicken Enchilada Bowl

Back when we were living in Compton, California, my mom used to make me enchiladas whenever I craved them. So when I have this healthy and heartfelt dish, I immediately think of her and it makes my soul smile.

**SERVES 2 or 3**
**PREP TIME:** 15 minutes
**COOK TIME:** 12 minutes

1 tablespoon olive oil
2 boneless, skinless chicken breasts
  (6 ounces each), cut into 1-inch chunks
¾ cup red enchilada sauce
1 (4-ounce) can chopped green chiles
¼ cup chopped yellow onion
1 cup cauliflower rice
1 cup chopped romaine lettuce

*Toppings*
½ avocado, pitted, peeled, and diced
1 jalapeño, finely chopped (ribs and seeds
  removed for less heat, if desired)
2 tablespoons shredded cheddar cheese
½ small Roma (plum) tomato, diced
1 tablespoon sour cream

1. In a large skillet, heat the oil over medium heat and cook the chicken until lightly browned but not cooked through, about 3 minutes.
2. Add the enchilada sauce, chiles, onion, and ¼ cup water and bring to a simmer. Cover and cook until the chicken is cooked through, about 3 minutes.
3. Meanwhile, place the cauliflower rice in a steamer set over a pan of simmering water, cover, and steam until the cauliflower is tender, about 5 minutes.
4. In a medium bowl, toss the lettuce with the steamed cauliflower and chicken and sauce. Serve with your choice of toppings.

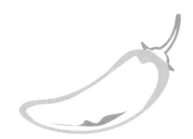

# Carne Asada with Chimichurri in Lettuce Wraps

I love when different Latino cultures come together to create a mouthwatering dish like this one. Mexico's carne asada infused with Argentina's chimichurri is so good, the minute you try this recipe you'll be hooked.

**SERVES 4**
**PREP TIME:** 10 minutes
**MARINATING TIME:** 2 hours to overnight
**COOK TIME:** 12 minutes

2 tablespoons avocado oil
2 tablespoons chopped cilantro
1 tablespoon fresh lime juice
1 tablespoon apple cider vinegar
1 teaspoon finely chopped garlic
1 teaspoon ground cumin
1 teaspoon dried oregano
1 teaspoon kosher salt
½ teaspoon cayenne pepper
½ teaspoon freshly ground black pepper
1-pound flank steak
Butter lettuce leaves
Chimichurri Sauce (page 126)

1. In a medium bowl, whisk together the oil, cilantro, lime juice, vinegar, garlic, cumin, oregano, salt, and cayenne and black peppers. Transfer the marinade to a shallow baking dish just large enough to hold the steak. Add the steak, cover, and refrigerate for at least 2 hours, or up to overnight, turning the steak a few times.

2. Remove the steak from the refrigerator 30 minutes before you plan on cooking and let it come to room temperature.

3. Heat a grill to medium and lightly oil the grates. Lift the steak out of the marinade and discard the marinade. Cook the steak until it reaches your desired degree of doneness, about 6 minutes per side for medium. (Do not do this inside on a grill pan as it will smoke.) Transfer the steak to a cutting board and let it cool for 10 minutes before slicing. Arrange the lettuce on a platter, top with the steak, drizzle with chimichurri sauce, and serve.

## Chimichurri Sauce

½ cup coarsely chopped parsley
4 cloves garlic, coarsely chopped
⅓ cup olive oil
¼ cup red wine vinegar
1 teaspoon finely grated lemon zest
1 teaspoon dried oregano
1 teaspoon red pepper flakes
½ teaspoon kosher salt

In a blender, pulse all the ingredients until well combined, but not pureed.

# Costillas de Puerco en Adobo con Ensalada de Nopales
## (Roasted Ribs with Cactus Salad)

The first vegetable I fell in love with as a little girl was the nopal, thanks to my *abuelita*. She'd sauté nopales with meat and red chiles or scramble them up with eggs and serve them for breakfast, explaining how good they were for me and how they'd help my digestion, and I was hooked. Nowadays I can have them with everything, including these ribs, or just on their own with a squeeze of lemon and a sprinkle of salt.

**SERVES 4**
**PREP TIME:** 15 minutes
**COOK TIME:** 3 hours

*For the rub and ribs*
2½ teaspoons kosher salt
2½ teaspoons paprika
1½ teaspoons ground cumin
1½ teaspoons Tajín
1 teaspoon oregano
1 teaspoon garlic powder
¾ teaspoon freshly ground black pepper
½ teaspoon thyme
½ teaspoon ground cinnamon
2½-pound rack baby back ribs

1. Preheat the oven to 300°F.
2. In a small bowl, combine all the rub ingredients and rub into both sides of the ribs. Wrap the ribs tightly in foil, place in a roasting pan, and bake until tender, about 2 hours.
3. Unwrap the ribs, discard the foil, and place the ribs back in the roasting pan. Cover with the sauce (recipe follows) and bake until the sauce is heated through, about 25 minutes.

(continued)

*For the sauce*

4 guajillo chiles, ribs and seeds removed

2 ancho chiles, ribs and seeds removed

1 teaspoon cumin seeds or ½ teaspoon
   ground cumin

1 teaspoon Mexican oregano

1 teaspoon dried thyme

½ teaspoon black peppercorns

1 bay leaf

¼ cup distilled white vinegar

1-inch soft cinnamon stick

2 cloves garlic, peeled

1 teaspoon kosher salt

1 cup chicken broth

1. In a large dry skillet warm the chiles for a few seconds over medium heat. Transfer to a bowl of hot water and let them soak until softened, about 20 minutes.

2. Lift the chiles from the hot water, transfer to a blender, and puree with the cumin, oregano, thyme, peppercorns, bay leaf, vinegar, cinnamon, garlic, salt, and chicken broth until smooth.

*For the nopales*

1 pound nopales, cleaned

2 Roma (plum) tomatoes, diced

1 small white onion, finely chopped

1 cup chopped cilantro

6 tablespoons fresh lemon juice

2 tablespoons olive oil

6 ounces crumbled ranchero cheese

½ teaspoon kosher salt

1. Wearing plastic gloves, and with a sharp knife, scrape or peel away the thorns on the nopales. Place the nopales on a cutting board, trim off about ¼ inch from the sides and bottoms, and cut them into ¼ × ½-inch pieces.

2. Place the nopales in a large pot and cover with cold water. Bring to a boil over high heat, then reduce the heat to medium and cook, skimming the slime that rises to the surface. Cook until the nopales are tender and no longer slimy, about 10 minutes. Drain and run them under cold water.

3. In a medium bowl, toss together the cooled and drained nopales, the tomatoes, onion, cilantro, lemon juice, oil, cheese, and salt. Serve alongside the ribs and sauce.

# Carne a la Tampiqueña with Roasted Zucchini

Carne a la tampiqueña is a super-popular Mexican dish at restaurants. Here's your chance to re-create a keto-friendly version at home and share it with your family and friends at the dinner table, while also allowing them to support your new lifestyle.

**SERVES 4**
**PREP TIME:** 20 minutes
**MARINATING TIME:** 30 minutes to overnight
**COOK TIME:** 25 minutes

1-pound skirt steak
½ teaspoon freshly ground black pepper
½ teaspoon garlic salt
1 pasilla chile
4 tablespoons olive oil
1 medium white onion, halved and thinly sliced
4 medium zucchini, halved lengthwise and sliced ½ inch thick
1 teaspoon kosher salt
½ teaspoon chili powder
½ teaspoon garlic powder
⅛ teaspoon cayenne pepper
1 tablespoon fresh lime juice
Crumbled Cotija cheese, for garnish
Fresh cilantro, for garnish

1. With a meat mallet or the bottom of a heavy skillet, pound the meat to ¼-inch thickness. Cut the steak into long pieces and sprinkle with ¼ teaspoon of the black pepper and the garlic salt.

2. On a grill or in a small skillet, toast the pasilla chile over medium heat for 2 minutes. Transfer to a bowl of warm water and let stand until softened, about 10 minutes. Remove the seeds and ribs and cut the chile into long strips.

3. In a small skillet, heat 1 tablespoon of the oil over medium heat. Add the onion and pasilla and sauté until the onion is crisp-tender, about 2 minutes.

4. In a medium bowl, toss the steak with the onion-pasilla mixture and 1 tablespoon of the remaining oil. Cover and refrigerate at least 30 minutes, or up to overnight.

5. Preheat the oven to 450°F. Line a rimmed sheet pan with parchment paper.

6. Toss the zucchini with the remaining 2 tablespoons oil, the salt, chili powder, garlic powder, the remaining ¼ teaspoon black pepper, and the cayenne. Transfer to the prepared sheet pan and bake until tender, about 20 minutes.

Drizzle with the lime juice and garnish with cheese and cilantro.

7. Heat the grill or a grill pan to medium and lightly oil the grates. Cook the steak, along with the onion-pasilla mixture, for about 30 seconds per side for medium-rare. Serve with the zucchini.

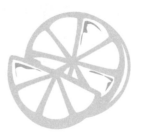

# Filete de Pescado with Cucumber and Cheese Salad

You can't get more summer on your plate than a cucumber and cheese salad accompanying a fillet of fish. This is a refreshing, nutritious, and light dish, perfect for warmer weather or for those nights when you're not feeling the need for a heavier meal. If your supermarket doesn't carry Cotija cheese, you can use feta cheese as a substitute to get that same crumbled, soft, and salty touch that makes this salad so special.

**SERVES 2**
**PREP TIME:** 10 minutes
**COOK TIME:** 10 minutes

3 Persian (mini) cucumbers, thinly sliced
1½ teaspoons plus ¼ cup olive oil
1 cup shredded Cotija cheese
2 tablespoons fresh lemon juice
1 teaspoon dried basil
1 teaspoon kosher salt
4 teaspoons fresh lime juice
1 teaspoon dried oregano
1 teaspoon chili powder
1 teaspoon garlic powder
½ teaspoon freshly ground black pepper
2 tilapia fillets (6 ounces each)
6 garlic cloves, peeled and crushed

1. In a medium bowl, toss the cucumbers with 1½ teaspoons of the oil, the cheese, lemon juice, basil, and ¼ teaspoon of the salt.

2. In a large bowl, whisk together the lime juice, oregano, chili powder, garlic powder, the remaining ¾ teaspoon salt, and the pepper. Add the fish, turning to coat.

3. In a large skillet, heat the remaining ¼ cup oil over medium-low heat, add the garlic, and cook until slightly golden, 3 to 4 minutes. Remove the garlic with a slotted spoon and discard.

4. Raise the heat to medium, add the fish, and cook until just cooked through, about 3 to 4 minutes per side. Divide the fish between two plates and serve with the cucumber salad.

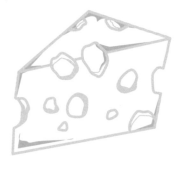

# Camarones a la Diabla with Mexican Kale Salad

Hot and spicy shrimp is absolutely the best of all worlds for me and Lorenzo. Every time we go to a seafood restaurant, we put in an order for camarones a la diabla. Any type of seafood with a kick makes me happy. I ate this dish a lot when I was a pescatarian, but back then my side of choice was white rice. Now we are mixing it up with this refreshing Mexican kale salad that I enjoy because I know I'm fueling my body with a healthy meal that also tastes amazing.

**SERVES 2**
**PREP TIME:** 15 minutes
**COOK TIME:** 30 minutes

2 medium tomatoes

6 tablespoons olive oil

2 chipotle peppers in adobo sauce, about 1 tablespoon

1 clove garlic, peeled

¼ teaspoon dried thyme

1 pound large shrimp (about 18), peeled and deveined

3 tablespoons lime juice

1 teaspoon kosher salt

¼ teaspoon freshly ground black pepper

⅓ cup diced white onion

1 tablespoon apple cider vinegar

1 tablespoon sugar-free maple syrup

½ teaspoon ancho chile powder

¼ teaspoon cayenne

1 (5-ounce) bag baby kale

1 pint cherry tomatoes, halved

¼ cup chopped cilantro

½ avocado, pitted, peeled, and diced

1 tablespoon hemp seeds

1. Preheat the oven to 400°F.

2. On a small rimmed sheet pan, roast the tomatoes until softened, about 20 minutes. When cool enough to handle, peel them. Transfer the peeled tomatoes to a blender and puree with 1 tablespoon of the oil, the chipotle peppers in adobo, garlic, and thyme.

3. Meanwhile, in a large bowl, toss the shrimp with 1 tablespoon of the lime juice, ½ teaspoon of the salt, and ⅛ teaspoon of the black pepper.

4. In a large skillet, heat 1 tablespoon of the oil over medium heat and sauté the onion until crisp-tender, about 3 minutes. Lift the shrimp from the marinade, add them to the skillet, and cook for 1 minute.

5. Add the pureed tomatoes, reduce the heat to low, and simmer until the shrimp are just cooked through, 2 to 3 minutes.

6. Meanwhile, in a large bowl, whisk together the remaining 2 tablespoons lime juice, the vinegar, maple syrup, ancho chile powder, cayenne, and the

remaining ½ teaspoon salt, ⅛ teaspoon
black pepper, and 4 tablespoons oil.
Add the kale, cherry tomatoes, cilantro,
avocado, and hemp seeds and toss to
combine. Divide the salad and shrimp
between two plates and serve.

# Mexican Meatsa

For those days when you just can't make up your mind, are hungry, and want a little bit of everything, this is your go-to dish. It's like a taco and a burger got married and had pizza as a kid. Plus, it's low carb and oh so satisfying.

SERVES 4
PREP TIME: 10 minutes
COOK TIME: 13 minutes

¾ pound (85% lean) ground beef

1 large egg

1 tablespoon taco seasoning

½ cup salsa

½ cup pitted black olives, sliced

1 jalapeño, seeds removed and coarsely chopped

1¼ cups shredded cheddar cheese

½ cup sour cream

¼ cup thinly sliced red onion

1 avocado, halved, pitted, peeled, and sliced

2 tablespoons chopped fresh cilantro

1 tablespoon fresh lime juice

¼ to ½ teaspoon red pepper flakes

1. Preheat the oven to 425°F. Line a rimmed sheet pan with parchment paper.

2. In a medium bowl, combine the beef, egg, and taco seasoning. Place the meat mixture on the prepared sheet pan and shape into a thin 9-inch round. Bake for 10 minutes or until the meat is no longer pink.

3. Top with the salsa, olives, jalapeño, and cheese and bake until the cheese has melted, about 3 minutes.

4. Remove the meat from the oven, top with the sour cream, onion, avocado, cilantro, lime juice, and red pepper flakes, and serve.

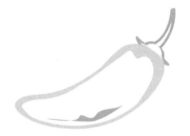

# Lemon Pepper Chicken Wings with Ranch Dressing

After church on Sundays, Lorenzo and I go home and unwind in front of the TV by watching football games, or any type of sport; although if the Cowboys are playing, it's even better! And we always share a plate of these delicious wings. I love putting a little extra pinch of lemon pepper in the ranch before dipping in my wing . . . it's amazing! This recipe is low carb and so good and quick and easy to make that I don't limit it to just Sundays or other game days; I usually have these babies twice a week.

**SERVES 2**
**PREP TIME:** 10 minutes
**COOK TIME:** 40 minutes

4 tablespoons ghee
1 tablespoon finely grated lemon zest
1 tablespoon fresh lemon juice
1 to 2 tablespoons freshly cracked black pepper
1½ teaspoons garlic salt
1 pound chicken wings, wing tips removed
½ cup grated Parmesan cheese
Ranch Dressing (page 101)

1. Preheat the oven to 400°F. Line a rimmed sheet pan with parchment paper and place a wire rack on top.

2. In a large bowl, combine the ghee, lemon zest, lemon juice, cracked pepper, and garlic salt. Add the chicken wings and toss to coat.

3. Place the wings on the rack, making sure they're spaced out evenly. Bake for 20 minutes on one side, then flip them over and bake until cooked through, about 20 minutes more. Transfer to a bowl. Add the Parmesan, tossing to coat, and serve with ranch dressing.

# Coconut Chicken Tenders

I grew up on chicken tenders. I ordered them all the time, mostly at fast food places. When I was a kid, we would usually go to Sizzlers after church and I didn't even have to look at the menu. I was all about those chicken strips, but I never knew how bad they were for me. That's why I love this healthy rendition of this childhood staple. It's got a similar consistency, and that touch of coconut makes them extra special. Love!

**SERVES 4**
**PREP TIME:** 10 minutes
**COOK TIME:** 20 minutes

1 large egg
1 cup unsweetened coconut flakes
½ cup cashew flour
¼ teaspoon kosher salt
¼ teaspoon freshly ground black pepper
¼ teaspoon garlic powder
⅛ teaspoon ground cinnamon
1 pound chicken tenders

1. Preheat the oven to 375°F. Line a rimmed sheet pan with parchment paper.

2. In a small shallow bowl, lightly beat the egg. In a medium bowl, combine the coconut (crushing it slightly if the flakes are large), cashew flour, salt, pepper, garlic powder, and cinnamon.

3. Dip the chicken tenders first into the egg and then into the coconut mixture, pressing them in. Place the tenders on the prepared sheet pan and bake for 10 minutes. Flip the tenders over and bake until the coating is crisp and the chicken is fully cooked, about 10 minutes more.

# Chicken Taquitos

Chicken taquitos bring me back to when I was between seven and ten years old. My mom would grab the leftovers of her *tinga de pollo* from the night before and turn them into chicken taquitos for us for the next day. We'd come home after school and heat them up in the microwave. To this day, these flavors still remind me of my mom.

**MAKES 3 TAQUITOS**
**PREP TIME:** 10 minutes
**COOK TIME:** 20 minutes

1 tablespoon olive oil

¼ cup finely chopped yellow onion

2 cloves garlic, finely chopped

½ teaspoon ground cumin

½ teaspoon chili powder

1½ cups shredded cooked chicken

⅓ cup red enchilada sauce

2 tablespoons chopped cilantro, plus more
  for garnish

2 cups shredded Mexican cheese blend

6 tablespoons sour cream, for garnish

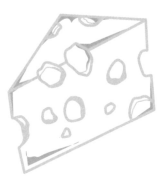

1. Preheat the oven to 375°F. Line 2 rimmed sheet pans with parchment paper.
2. In a medium skillet, heat the oil over medium heat. Add the onion and sauté until tender, about 3 minutes. Add the garlic, cumin, and chili powder and sauté for 1 minute longer.
3. Add the chicken, enchilada sauce, and cilantro to the skillet and bring to a simmer. Cook, until the chicken is heated through, about 2 minutes.
4. Meanwhile, make 3 equal mounds of cheese on each prepared sheet pan, placing them 3 inches apart, flatten them slightly, and bake until melted and golden brown around the edges, 8 to 10 minutes.
5. Allow the cheese to cool for 2 minutes. Place 2½ tablespoons of the chicken on the top third of each cheese round and roll them up.
6. Garnish with cilantro and the sour cream and serve.

# Broiled Salmon with Arugula Salad

Another salmon recipe to boost your healthy, good-for-you fat intake, keep you satisfied, and help you hit all your macros in one go. And the lemony, citrusy arugula salad is the perfect way to complete this delicious meal.

**SERVES 4**
**PREP TIME:** 10 minutes
**COOK TIME:** 5 minutes

4 teaspoons grainy mustard

2 cloves garlic, finely minced

1 tablespoon finely minced shallot

1½ teaspoons finely chopped fresh thyme, plus more for garnish

1½ teaspoons finely chopped fresh rosemary

4 tablespoons fresh lemon juice

Kosher salt and freshly ground black pepper to taste

4 skinless salmon fillets (5 ounces each)

4 lemon slices

1½ tablespoons olive oil

4½ cups baby arugula

¼ cup freshly shaved Parmesan

1. Heat the broiler on medium with the rack 6 inches from the heat. Line a rimmed sheet pan with foil.

2. In a small bowl, stir together the mustard, garlic, shallots, thyme, rosemary, and 2 tablespoons of the lemon juice. Season with salt and pepper.

3. Dip each salmon fillet into the bowl, place them on the prepared sheet pan, and spoon any of the remaining mustard mixture over the top. Place a lemon slice on each fillet and broil until cooked to desired degree of doneness (timing will vary depending upon the thickness of the fillets), about 5 minutes for medium-rare.

4. In a medium bowl, whisk together the remaining 2 tablespoons lemon juice and the oil; season with salt and pepper. Add the arugula, tossing to coat. Scatter the Parmesan over the salad and serve with the salmon garnished with thyme.

# Chili for the Soul

Chili makes me think of winter; it's my comfort food for the soul. This recipe is heavenly because it makes me feel the same way as regular chili minus the bloat and guilt. It's what I turn to when I want to eat something super savory and indulging on a cold and rainy day.

**SERVES 4**
**PREP TIME:** 10 minutes
**COOK TIME:** 25 minutes

3 slices bacon, halved crosswise

¼ medium yellow onion, finely chopped

2 celery stalks, finely chopped

1 green bell pepper, coarsely chopped

½ cup thinly sliced baby bella mushrooms

2 cloves garlic, finely chopped

1 pound (85% lean) ground beef

1 tablespoon chili powder

1 tablespoon smoked paprika

1 teaspoon ground cumin

1 teaspoon dried oregano

1 teaspoon kosher salt

½ teaspoon freshly ground black pepper

1 cup beef broth

¼ cup shredded cheddar cheese

4 teaspoons sour cream

¼ cup thinly sliced scallions

1 avocado, halved, pitted, peeled, and sliced

1. In a large skillet, cook the bacon over medium-low heat until it has rendered its fat and is crisp, about 5 minutes. With a slotted spoon, transfer the bacon to a paper-towel-lined plate; leave the bacon fat in the skillet. Crumble the bacon.

2. Add the onion, celery, bell pepper, and mushrooms to the skillet and cook over medium heat until crisp-tender, about 5 minutes. Add the garlic and cook for another minute.

3. Add the beef, chili powder, paprika, cumin, oregano, salt, and pepper and cook, stirring frequently, until the beef is no longer pink, about 5 minutes.

4. Add the broth, bring to a simmer, cover, and cook until the liquid has been absorbed, about 7 minutes.

5. To serve, divide the beef among four bowls and top with the bacon, cheese, sour cream, scallions, and avocado.

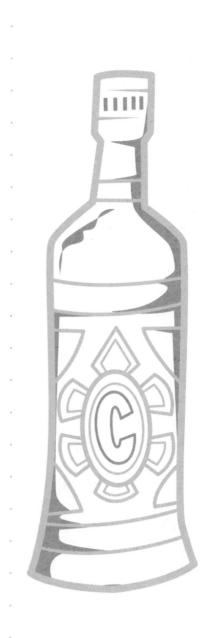

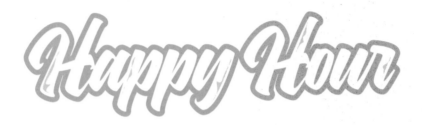

# Happy Hour

*A little alcohol never hurt nobody. . . . These recipes are perfect when, once in a while, you need a little something-something to unwind from a long day. Make yourself a Paloma Blanca and just chill, or throw an Ay Mojito, Qué Rico party with your girls. Just make sure you keep it at one or two drinks per week max, enough to get you feeling nice without throwing you offtrack.*

## SHOPPING LIST

### Alcohol
light beer

tequila

vodka

### Soda, Juice, and Citrus
Clamato juice

coconut club soda

grapefruit-flavored sparkling water

grapefruit juice

limes

### Miscellaneous
lakanto syrup

mint leaves

orange extract

pink Himalayan salt

stevia

# Ay Mojito, Qué Rico

Any time I have this drink, it immediately reminds me of my honeymoon with Lorenzo in Puerto Rico. It takes me back to lying next to him, beachside, without a care in the world, and dozing off to the sound of the ocean waves and breeze.

SERVES 1

PREP TIME: 5 minutes

4 fresh mint leaves

2 teaspoons granulated stevia

2 tablespoons fresh lime juice

2 ounces (¼ cup) vodka

Ice cubes or crushed ice

Coconut club soda

Lime slice, for garnish

In a cocktail shaker, muddle the mint leaves with a muddler or wooden spoon. Add the stevia and lime juice and mix until the stevia has dissolved. Add the vodka and ice and shake well. Strain into a glass, top with the club soda, and garnish with the lime slice.

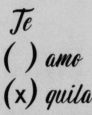

# Te
# ( ) amo
# (x) quila

I am an outright *tequilera* . . . I can drink ten shots like a man and still stay standing. What I love about it is that it's clean, straight to the point, and gets the job done. When Sarah told me that I could still drink tequila while adopting this keto-friendly lifestyle, it was music to my ears. I mean, I drink tequila to wind down and I drink shots on stage with my fans. If I'm at a party, the first thing I will order is a tequila beyond any other drink on the menu. And now I love sharing this drink with Sarah. She's not just the one who taught me how to order keto-friendly drinks at the bar, we've also shared tequila and some memorable moments together. If you like it spicy and tangy, like me, add Tajín to the rim for an extra kick!

**SERVES 1**
**PREP TIME:** 5 minutes

Ice cubes
2 ounces (¼ cup) tequila
2 tablespoons lakanto syrup
2 tablespoons fresh lime juice
½ teaspoon orange extract
Lime wedge

Fill a cocktail shaker with ice and add the tequila, lakanto syrup, lime juice, and orange extract and shake until well chilled. Strain into a glass and top with the lime wedge.

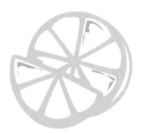

# Paloma Blanca

There is a tequila drink out there called Paloma, but Sarah and I gave it a little grapefruit twist to make it our own. "Paloma Blanca" is actually the title of my first single, a song dedicated to my mom. It's bittersweet because although it was my first single and a tribute to my mom, the recording wasn't up to par with what I was hoping to do as an artist. It wasn't ready to come out, I know this now, but at the time I received bucketloads of criticism because of it. However, to this day, I try to sidestep that judgment and focus on why I wrote that song—it was for my mom, a message to her from deep in my heart after she passed away, and nothing and no one will take that away from me. As the song's chorus says, *"Vuela alto, vuela libre"* (fly high and free, so sip and enjoy!).

**SERVES 1**

**PREP TIME:** 5 minutes

Pink Himalayan salt

Ice cubes

¼ cup fresh grapefruit juice

2 ounces (¼ cup) tequila

1½ to 2 tablespoons fresh lime juice

Grapefruit-flavored sparkling water

1. Place pink salt on a small flat plate. Moisten the rim of a glass with water and twist it in the salt to coat.

2. Fill a cocktail shaker with ice and add the grapefruit juice, tequila, and lime juice and shake until well chilled. Strain into the prepared glass and top with some sparkling water.

# Michelada

Beer on Chi-Keto? Hells yeah, as long as it's light. I love having this drink on Sunday Fundays when I'm spending time with my family and friends while having aguachile or carne asada on the grill. You can never go wrong with this refreshing and savory drink!

SERVES 1
PREP TIME: 5 minutes

6 ounces (¾ cup) light beer, chilled
3 ounces (6 tablespoons) Clamato juice, chilled
2 teaspoons fresh lime juice
½ teaspoon Tapatío hot sauce, or more to taste
Tajín to taste
Ice cubes, if desired

In a tall glass, stir together the beer, Clamato juice, lime juice, Tapatío, and Tajín. Add ice, if desired.

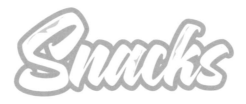

# Snacks

*I know it's a struggle when we are trying to look like a snack while craving snacks. Come on, you don't think I miss making a stop at the local elotero stand? But, priorities, baby! The next time your fiending for an elote, try the Cauliflower Elote (page 149). And if your sweet tooth is whispering sweet nothings in your ear, then go for the Mexican Hot Chocolate Pudding (page 157) and call it a day. Just keep it to no more than one snack between breakfast and lunch and another between lunch and dinner and you will be golden.*

## Chingona Tip

For those hectic, on-the-go days when time to prep snacks is limited, simply grab a zip-top resealable bag, fill it with a handful of nuts and seeds, and put it in your purse. That way, if you're stuck in traffic or running from one meeting to the next, you'll have a handy snack to help you power through to your next meal. I got you, girl.

## SHOPPING LIST

avocado
baby spinach
bacon
cauliflower
chia seeds
cilantro
cream cheese
cucumbers
eggs
fresh blueberries
fresh strawberries
ghee
ham (1-ounce slices)

heavy cream
jalapeños
limes
Mexican crema
Mölli Culiacan Chamoy sauce
roasted unsalted cashews
scallions
shredded cheddar cheese
shredded Cotija cheese
stevia
tomato
unsweetened cocoa powder
unsweetened coconut milk

# Cauliflower Elote

Now you know I couldn't have a cookbook without an *elote* (Mexican street corn) recipe! It's another one of my childhood favorites. This takes me back to when we lived in Long Beach and I was at my *abuelita*'s house. Any time I heard the *elotero*'s horn ringing on the block, even if I was upstairs watching TV, I'd come rushing down and out to his cart and ask him for an "*elote con todo*" (corn with everything on it . . . and extra chile). I'd walk back into the house, digging into my cup, and my mom would say, "Don't eat that, *te vas a poner bien gorda!*" But I didn't care if it would make me fat or not; I would eat it almost every day back then. Sometimes I'd lag behind after school with my friends just to catch the *elotero*—the same guy who served our street for years—because I knew he walked down that block on certain days. I was such an *elote* addict that I knew what time he usually walked by and at what corners he liked to park his cart for a while.

**SERVES 3 or 4**
**PREP TIME:** 10 minutes
**COOK TIME:** 45 minutes

1 large cauliflower (about 2½ pounds)

3 tablespoons avocado oil

1⅛ teaspoons kosher salt

5 tablespoons Cotija cheese

3 tablespoons mayonnaise

2 tablespoons Mexican crema

1 tablespoon chopped cilantro

1 tablespoon fresh lime juice

1 tablespoon Tajín, plus more for garnish if desired

⅛ teaspoon cayenne pepper, plus more for garnish if desired

¼ cup sliced scallions, for garnish

1. Preheat the oven to 375°F. Line a rimmed sheet pan with parchment paper.

2. Core the cauliflower and cut it into florets. Transfer the florets to a large bowl and toss with the oil and 1 teaspoon of the salt. Dump the cauliflower onto the prepared sheet pan in a single layer and roast, turning the cauliflower once or twice, until tender, about 45 minutes.

3. Meanwhile, in a large bowl, combine the cheese, mayonnaise, crema, cilantro, lime juice, Tajín, cayenne, and the remaining ⅛ teaspoon salt. Add the cauliflower and toss to coat. Garnish with the scallions and more Tajín or cayenne pepper, if desired, and serve.

# Pepinos Locos

These are so mouthwatering, refreshing, crunchy, and spicy that they drive me *loca* because they're so good! What can I say? Let's just put chamoy on everything from now on!

MAKES 12 PIECES (2 per serving)
PREP TIME: 10 minutes

3 large cucumbers, peeled, halved lengthwise, and seeded

⅓ cup Mölli Culiacan Chamoy sauce, plus more for topping if desired

⅓ cup Tajín, plus more for topping if desired

1 cup roasted unsalted cashews, coarsely chopped

Fresh lime juice

1. Halve the cucumbers crosswise. Pour the chamoy sauce onto one small plate and the Tajíin onto another. Dip the cut sides of each cucumber into the chamoy sauce and then into the Tajín. Turn the cucumbers cut side up onto a platter and spoon the cashews onto each one.

2. If desired, top with lime juice and a little more chamoy sauce and Tajín.

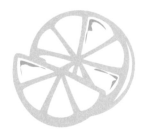

# Ham and Cheesy Egg Rollup

Pre-workout or post-workout it's my favorite anytime/anywhere snack. Easy and quick!

MAKES 4 ROLLUPS (2 per serving)
PREP TIME: 5 minutes
COOK TIME: 10 minutes

2 large eggs

1 teaspoon garlic powder

¼ teaspoon kosher salt

Freshly ground black pepper to taste

1 teaspoon ghee

½ cup shredded cheddar cheese

½ cup baby spinach

½ small tomato, chopped

4 (1-ounce) slices ham

1. Heat the broiler on low with the rack 6 inches from the heat.

2. In a small bowl, lightly beat the eggs with the garlic powder, salt, and pepper.

3. In a medium nonstick skillet, heat the ghee over medium heat. Add the egg mixture, cheese, spinach, and tomato and cook, stirring constantly, until the eggs are set but still soft, about 4 minutes.

4. Arrange the slices of ham on a serving platter and top each with 2 to 3 tablespoons of the cooked eggs and roll up the ham from one of the short ends.

5. Place the rollups seam side down on a small rimmed sheet pan or broiler pan and broil until the ham is lightly crisped, about 5 minutes. Divide between two plates and serve.

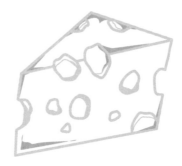

# Bacon-Wrapped Jalapeño Poppers

Jalapeño poppers are the bomb, but they are loaded with carbs. So this is a refreshing keto-friendly alternative that will hit the flavorful notes you have come to expect from a good popper. It's a satisfying and spicy snack, just like me. 😉

**MAKES 20 POPPERS (4 per serving)**
**PREP TIME:** 10 minutes
**COOK TIME:** 20 minutes

10 jalapeños, halved lengthwise, ribs and
  seeds removed
4 ounces cream cheese, softened
¼ cup shredded cheddar cheese
1 teaspoon paprika
10 slices bacon, halved lengthwise

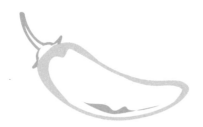

1. Preheat the oven to 375°F. Line a rimmed sheet pan with parchment paper.
2. Slice the stem end and bottom off each jalapeño.
3. In a small bowl, mix together the cream cheese, cheddar, and paprika. With a spoon, divide the cheese mixture among the jalapeño halves. Wrap a bacon half around each jalapeño half.
4. Place the bacon-wrapped jalapeños, leaving space between them, on the prepared sheet pan and bake until the bacon is fully cooked, about 20 minutes. Serve hot.

# Turkey-Wrapped Mozzarella Stick

Another awesome game-day snack to steer you clear of junk food while still keeping you satisfied. It's also a great post-workout snack.

SERVES 1

1 slice deli turkey
1 mozzarella stick

Wrap the turkey slice around the mozzarella stick and enjoy.

# Keto Refried Beans

SERVES 6 (²⁄₃ cup per serving)
PREP TIME: 10 minutes
COOK TIME: 20 minutes

2 tablespoons olive oil

½ cup finely chopped yellow onion

2 cloves garlic, thinly sliced

2 (15-ounce) cans black soybeans,
  drained and rinsed

1 tablespoon ground cumin

1 teaspoon kosher salt

½ teaspoon freshly ground black pepper

1 (4-ounce) Mexican (fresh) chorizo,
  casing removed

12 tablespoons shredded Monterey Jack
  or Cotija cheese

1. In a large skillet, heat 1 tablespoon of the oil over medium-low heat. Add the onion and garlic and cook, stirring frequently until the onion has softened, about 7 minutes.

2. Transfer the onion and garlic to a food processor. Add the beans, cumin, salt, pepper, and remaining tablespoon oil and process until smooth.

3. Meanwhile heat the same skillet over medium heat, add the chorizo and cook, stirring to break up the meat, until no longer pink, about 2 minutes. Add the bean mixture and cook, stirring frequently until piping hot and bubbly, about 8 minutes. Divide the mixture among 6 plates. Sprinkle each with 2 tablespoons of cheese and serve.

# Fruit Cup with Tajín

You know you're Latina when you add lime juice and Tajín to your fruit! If you've never tried this combo before, what are you waiting for? After your first bite, the burst of flavors will have you wanting more.

**SERVES 1**
**PREP TIME:** 5 minutes

2 tablespoons fresh lime juice, or more to taste

1½ teaspoons Tajín, or more to taste

1 tablespoon chia seeds

½ cup raspberries

½ cup sliced strawberries

In a small bowl, whisk together the lime juice, Tajín, and chia seeds. Add the fruit and toss to combine. You can always add more Tajín and lime juice, but do not add more fruit.

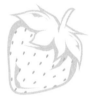

# Chia Seed Arroz con Leche

*Arroz con leche* is such a huge staple dessert in Latin America that it even has its own nursery rhyme! When Sarah and I were talking about how this recipe had to be in this book, she actually told me that it even resembles a Middle Eastern dessert she grew up having as a kid called *gatnabour*. Her *abuelita* used to make it for her each time she visited. Nothing like finding such similarities among different cultures, showing us how united we all really are. Bonus: chia seeds are high in fiber, which make them your BFF when it comes time to go to the restroom.

**MAKES 2 CUPS (1 cup per serving)**
**PREP TIME:** 5 minutes
**REFRIGERATING TIME:** Overnight

1 cup unsweetened coconut milk
½ cup heavy cream
⅓ cup chia seeds
1 teaspoon stevia
2 teaspoons vanilla extract
1 teaspoon ground cinnamon
Small pinch of sea salt

1. In a medium bowl, stir together all the ingredients. Let stand for 5 minutes, then stir again. Cover and refrigerate. Or, if you've got one, transfer the mixture to a mason jar, cover, and refrigerate overnight. The longer it sits in the refrigerator, the thicker it will get.
2. Have 1 cup for a serving.

# Mexican Hot Chocolate Pudding

Every spoonful of this pudding reminds me of the Abuelita brand's Mexican-style hot chocolate and my own *abuelita*. When I went to my *abuelita*'s house, I knew she kept the Abuelita chocolate tablets in her kitchen cabinets, so when no one was looking, I'd sneak in, unwrap the bar, and take a bite out of it, then put it away. Later, if my sweet tooth kicked in again, I'd tiptoe into the kitchen and take another bite or two. It was sooo good! Then, when she would reach for the Abuelita chocolate, she'd open it and find my teeth marks all over it! So I needed to have something to satisfy this craving, and this pudding sure does the job!

**SERVES 1**

**PREP TIME:** 5 minutes

½ avocado, pitted, peeled, and cut into chunks

2 tablespoons unsweetened coconut milk

1 tablespoon erythritol

1½ teaspoons unsweetened cocoa powder

1½ teaspoons ground cinnamon

¼ teaspoon vanilla extract

Pinch of cayenne pepper

Pinch of stevia

Pinch of pink Himalayan salt, if desired

In a small food processor or blender, puree all the ingredients until smooth. Top the pudding off with a pinch of pink Himalayan salt, if you like.

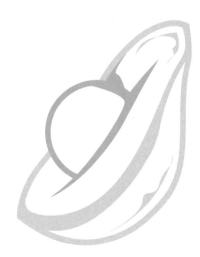

# Chocolate Strawberry Mousse

One of my all-time favorite desserts is chocolate-covered strawberries. If you dip them in dark chocolate, it's actually okay to have a couple while doing keto. But this dessert takes that to another level, expanding that simple snack into a delicious dessert that will help you calm your sugar craving in a heartbeat.

**SERVES 2**
**PREP TIME:** 5 minutes

1 cup heavy cream
2 tablespoons unsweetened cocoa powder
2 tablespoons erythritol
1 teaspoon vanilla extract
5 fresh strawberries, hulled and halved
Whipped cream

1. In the bowl of an electric mixer, with the whisk attachment, beat the cream, cocoa powder, erythritol, and vanilla until thick, about 3 minutes.
2. Fold in the strawberries, divide between 2 bowls, and top with whipped cream.

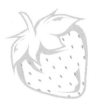

# Berries and Cream

Who said we can't have fruit on keto? All we need to do is stick to the low-sugar varieties, such as the blueberries and strawberries in this recipe. Combined with the vanilla whipped cream, it's just like a little slice of heaven. Can't live without it!

SERVES 2
PREP TIME: 5 minutes

⅔ cup heavy cream

¼ teaspoon vanilla extract

½ cup fresh blueberries

½ cup fresh strawberries, hulled and thickly sliced

1 teaspoon chia seeds

1. In the bowl of an electric mixer with the whisk attachment, beat the cream on medium to soft peaks. Then beat in the vanilla.

2. Transfer the cream to a serving bowl, fold in the blueberries and strawberries, sprinkle over the chia seeds, and serve.

# FIVE

# The 12 Essential Exercises
# for a Chingona's Body

These are the exercises that will help keep you strong and fit throughout your Chi-Keto journey. The weekly workouts from chapter 3 are broken down here into twelve essential exercises with variations to make them a little more challenging as you progress and get stronger.

Working out makes me feel so much better physically, mentally, and emotionally. Whether I'm going through the feels or had a tough day, I use this time as a form of escape. There's just something about sweating all the stress away that puts me in the best mood. This doesn't mean it's easy. You will struggle, but just don't quit. Sometimes you will wonder, *Why the heck am I doing this?* Because it hurts like crazy at first. It's uncomfortable. Your muscles are screaming for you to stop because they're not used to being moved like that. Hey, I'll admit it, there are days I'd much rather skip my work-out, snuggle up in my blanket, and watch a movie with a tub of mint chocolate chip ice cream. But I've learned that the mind is a powerful thing. Sometimes you've got to get up, look in the mirror, and remind yourself that you are a boss bee. And that you are stronger than your excuses.

One of the most important things in this journey is having a support system. Whether it's a friend whom you've made a pact with to work out together and keep each other accountable, or your *loca* personal trainer who shows up at your house at six in the morning with full-blown energy and a workout/twerkout playlist. Luckily for me, Sarah is both. Her method is simple and straight to the point, just how I like it. What I love about her routines is that you can do them at home or on the road because there's no need for crazy equipment or a gym membership. All you need to get started is a couple of dumbbells that are challenging enough for you to break a sweat and a resistance band set. Easy, right? There is no room for excuses.

Before you get started, please read the following instructions carefully:

- All exercises can be performed at the gym or at home. The only equipment needed is dumbbells and ankle resistance bands.
- Start with five-pound weights. If they become too easy, try to increase the weights you use by two to five pounds a week. If they become too heavy, regress to a more comfortable weight until you're ready for the next challenge.
- Make sure you have eaten a well-balanced meal or snack forty-five minutes to one hour before you start your workout.
- Begin your workout with a seven-minute warm-up with your choice of jumping jacks, jogging in place, or jumping rope.
- After your warm-up, begin the day's workout. Do one set of repetitions of each exercise in the daily workout plan, then repeat the round until you have completed all three sets. Record and keep track of your weights and repetitions performed.
- Form is essential to avoid injuries. Make sure you pay close attention to each exercise's instructions and, when available, refer to the accompanying photo.
- If any exercise or recommended repetition becomes too difficult, don't exert yourself to complete it as instructed. Do it at your own pace and don't forget to hydrate with water.
- If at any point you feel lightheaded, dizzy, faint, or have any sort of pain, please stop. Burning muscles are normal, pain is not.
- Try your best not to sit down between exercises. Instead, remain on your feet and walk or dance around until you're ready to move on to the following exercise.
- Space out the three weekly workouts with one day off in between. For example: do Workout 1 on Monday, Workout 2 on Wednesday, and Workout 3 on Friday. You can also choose Tuesday, Thursday, and Saturday, or whatever fits your schedule best.
- Make sure to get thirty to forty-five minutes of daily cardio. Remember: your heart is a muscle; if you do not work it out, it does not work for you.
- After completing your workout, stretch and replenish your body with a Chi-Keto meal or snack.

- Once you've completed the 21-day workout plan, head over to bootyfitworkout .com for more exercise guides and fitness routines to follow. Get ready, Sarah's all about booty-focused workouts!

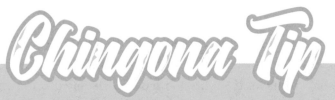

*Let's keep it real: there will be days when you are just going to want to skip a workout. Your PMS cramps may be so bad that you need to stay curled up in a ball in bed. Or you may wake up with a nasty flu. Or you may have stayed up all night to make a deadline and decide to sacrifice your daily workout for an extra hour of sleep the next morning. We all have those days. So go ahead and take that day to rest and recharge, or opt for a jog or a dance session in your room, but get right back on track the following morning.*

*It takes small changes to make a big change, mama.*
*You are capable; you just have to stay consistent!*

### ESSENTIAL EXERCISE 1: GLUTE BRIDGES

Lie faceup on the floor, with your knees bent and feet hip-width apart and flat on the ground. Place your arms to the sides of your body. Lift your glutes off the ground, hold at the top for 3 seconds, then slowly drop them back to the ground. This is one repetition.

*Variation for Week 2, Workout 1:* **Banded Glute Bridges**

Place a resistance band just above your knees. Set up for a glute bridge and perform as described above.

*Variation for Week 3, Workout 1:* **Glute Bridges to Chest Presses**

Lie faceup on the floor and set up for a glute bridge as described above. Grab one dumbbell in each hand and hold them up with your elbows resting on the ground in a starting chest press position. As you lift your glutes off the ground also extend your arms toward the ceiling into a chest press, hold for 3 seconds, then slowly drop your glutes and arms back to the starting position on the ground.

## ESSENTIAL EXERCISE 2: BANDED BICEP CURLS

With your feet firmly planted on the ground and with a nice straight back, stand on the middle of a resistance band with your feet hip-width apart. The wider you stand, the more resistance you will have. If there's too much resistance, bring your feet closer together to decrease it. Pushing your shoulders back and engaging your core, extend your arms straight down next to your body and, holding the handles of the band in each hand with your palms facing up, bend your arms at the elbows and curl them up into a bicep curl. As you perform each repetition, keep a controlled speed so you get full flexion and extension of your arms, and make sure your elbows remain close to your body. If you find your torso moving back and forth, then you might want to reduce the resistance to make sure your body is still. The only parts of your body that should be moving are your arms.

*Variation for Week 2, Workout 1:* Dumbbell Bicep Curls

Perform bicep curls as described above, with one dumbbell in each hand instead of the resistance band handles.

*Variation for Week 3, Workout 1:* Alternating Bicep Curls

Set up for bicep curls, but instead of bringing both arms up, curl one arm up, lower it, then curl the other arm up and lower it. This is one repetition.

## ESSENTIAL EXERCISE 3: BANDED SQUATS
## (WITH LOOP RESISTANCE BAND)

Place a resistance band just above your knees with your feet hip-width apart and toes facing straight ahead. To perform a squat, squeeze your core, push your booty out as if you were about to sit on a chair, and drop into your squat, making sure your knees are aligned with your ankles and you are pushing your knees against the band. Press your heels into the ground to maintain proper form. If needed, lift your toes slightly off the ground to force your body into the correct position. Return to the starting position and repeat to complete one set.

*Variation for Week 2, Workout 1:* Dumbbell Squats

Stand with your feet hip-width apart. Grab a dumbbell in each hand, bend your elbows, and bring your hands to your shoulders, resting the dumbbells there and keeping your elbows close to your body throughout the set. Perform your squat as described above, return to the starting position, and repeat.

*Variation for Week 3, Workout 1:* Squats to Shoulder Presses

Stand with your feet hip-width apart with one dumbbell in each hand, elbows bent, and your hands and dumbbells on top of your shoulders. Drop into a squat, come up, then extend your arms all the way to the ceiling into a shoulder press. Bring your arms down to your shoulders and repeat.

## ESSENTIAL EXERCISE 4: PLANK

Get on the floor in pushup position. Your arms should be extended straight beneath you with your hands directly aligned with your shoulders. Your legs should extend straight back with feet hip-width apart. Engage your core and form a straight line with your body, making sure to keep a straight back at all times. Keep a neutral neck. If you feel yourself dipping, tighten up your core and fix your form so as to not strain your lower back. Also avoid doing the opposite and bending at the waist with your booty in the air. To reap the greatest benefits, it's all about maintaining that sturdy, straight, plank-shaped line in your body.

## ESSENTIAL EXERCISE 5: STAGNANT LUNGES

Step ahead onto your right foot. Your right knee should be aligned with that ankle. Always make sure this alignment is spot-on to avoid hyperflexing those muscles, and don't be afraid to stop and correct your form while doing the repetitions. Place your hands on your hips and, while keeping your front right leg nice and stable, drop your back left leg into a lunge, then bring it back up to the starting position, allowing that back leg to do all the work. Finish the repetitions with your left leg, then step back, switch legs, bringing your left foot forward, and lunge with your right leg. When you are done with these repetitions, you will have completed one set.

*Variation for Week 2, Workout 2:* **Alternating Lunges**

Step forward in your lunge position, lunge, then step back to the starting position and step forward with the other leg, lunge, and step back. This equals one repetition. Continue until you complete the set.

*Variation for Week 3, Workout 2:* **Stagnant Lunges to Bicep Curls**

Grab one dumbbell in each hand and extend your arms down next to your body, palms facing inward. Step forward into your stagnant lunge position. Perform a lunge, then bend your elbows and curl your arms up into a bicep curl, keeping your elbows close to your body, extend back down, and push up with your leg to the starting position. Complete the repetitions on one leg, then switch and repeat with the other leg. This will conclude one set.

## ESSENTIAL EXERCISE 6: PUSH-UPS

Get into a plank position, keeping a straight and flat back with your arms extended beneath you and perfectly aligned with your shoulders. If you're doing a modified push-up, simply drop your knees to the floor and cross your feet but continue to maintain that nice, flat back and aligned arms throughout the exercise. Bend your arms at the elbows and bring your chest down as close to the ground as possible, keeping that straight, flat back at all times, then push your torso back up to the starting position and repeat until you complete your set. You may not get your chest very close to the floor when you first start, and that's okay. Don't break your form, just go deeper. Patience, you will get there eventually.

## ESSENTIAL EXERCISE 7: BACK ROWS

Stand with your feet hip-width apart and a slight bend in your knees. Grab one dumbbell in each hand and bend forward at your hips so that your chest is parallel to the floor, your arms are hanging beneath you straight from the shoulders, palms facing inward, and your booty is pushed back with your weight on your heels to maintain proper form. Relax and push your shoulders back, then squeeze your upper back, bend your elbows, and slowly pull them up to the sky, keeping your arms close to your body at all times. Hold for 2 seconds, then slowly bring your arms down to the starting position, engaging your core at all times so as to not lose your form, and repeat. If you perform your back rows too quickly, you will lose engagement of your back and instead start working your biceps, defying the purpose of this exercise. Remember to keep your eyes on the ground and make sure to relax your neck and shoulders while doing each set.

### Variation for Week 2, Workout 2: Single-Arm Back Rows

Get in your back-row position, but this time stagger your stance, bringing your right leg in front of you and the left leg behind you, keeping your knees slightly bent, with your chest parallel to the ground as with your regular back row. Now simply perform a back row pulling only your right arm back while keeping your left arm in the starting position. Return your right arm to the starting position and continue to repeat the exercise with your right arm. Then switch legs and arms and complete the repetitions on the left side to finish one set.

### Variation for Week 3, Workout 2: Plank Rows

Get into your plank position with a dumbbell next to each hand. Grab one dumbbell with your right hand, keeping your shoulders, back, and neck neutral, and bend your arm as you raise your elbow to the sky, keeping your arm close to your torso at all times and a strong core. Keep your hips parallel to the floor. Bring your arm down, release the dumbbell, return to your standard plank, and repeat the movement with your left arm. This equals one repetition. Keep going to complete the set!

### ESSENTIAL EXERCISE 8: CRUNCHES

Lie flat on the ground, facing up, with your knees bent and your feet hip-width apart and flat on the floor. Make sure your lower back remains flat on the ground at all times to avoid arching, which can hurt your back. Place your hands behind your head to protect your neck, elbows out to the sides as far back as they can go, and keep your chin up. Tighten your core and curl up, peeling your head, neck, and shoulder blades off the floor to perform one crunch. Return to the starting position and repeat to complete one set. If you notice your elbows creeping up to your ears, push them back to correct your form.

## ESSENTIAL EXERCISE 9: MOUNTAIN CLIMBERS

Get into your standard plank position, remembering to always keep that straight and flat line along your back and legs, with your hands directly beneath your shoulders, and a nice strong core. Bring your right knee up and tap it against your right elbow (or as far as you can go), then bring it back to starting plank position and repeat with your left knee tapping your left elbow. Bring your left knee back to the starting position to complete one repetition. Continue until you finish your set.

## ESSENTIAL EXERCISE 10: SHOULDER PRESSES

Stand with your feet hip-width apart, a slight bend in your knees, and one dumbbell in each hand. Bring your arms up, parallel to the floor and aligned horizontally with your shoulders, and bend your elbows at a 90-degree angle so your palms are facing forward and your fists are pointing upward. Keeping a straight back and your core engaged, extend both arms to the ceiling, bring them both back to the starting position, and repeat until you complete your set.

### Variation for Week 2, Workout 3: Alternating Shoulder Presses

Set up in the starting position for a shoulder press, as described above, but now extend only your right arm to the ceiling. Once you return it to the starting position, extend your left arm up and back down to complete one repetition. Continue until you finish your set.

### Variation for Week 3, Workout 3: Squats to Shoulder Presses

Stand in a starting squat position, with dumbbells in your hands and placed on top of your shoulders. Drop into your squat, come up, then extend your arms to the sky to perform one shoulder press. Return your arms to the starting position and repeat the exercise until you complete your set.

## ESSENTIAL EXERCISE 11: GLUTE KICKBACKS

Get on your hands and knees, placing your hands directly beneath your shoulders and your knees hip-width apart. Keeping a nice, flat back, engage your core and kick one leg back, keeping it bent at the knee so that the heel of your foot is facing the sky. Hold for 2 seconds, then slowly bring it down and repeat with your other leg.

*Variation for Weeks 2 and 3, Workout 3:* **Banded Glute Kickbacks**

Grab a resistance band and, holding the handles in each hand, hook the middle of the band on the arch of your right foot. Get into your glute kickback position and, maintaining a flat back and engaged core, push the band back with your right foot and extend your leg out straight. Return to the starting position and repeat with the same leg. Complete the repetitions on your right leg, then switch to your left leg and repeat to complete one set.

## ESSENTIAL EXERCISE 12: TRICEP DIPS

Stand with your feet hip-width apart and a slight bend in your knees. With a dumbbell in each hand, bend at the hip to position your chest parallel to the floor, arms bent at the elbows and placed close to your body with your hands near your shoulders. Engage your core to maintain a nice, flat back, and push your forearms back, always keeping your elbows close to your body. Return to the starting position and repeat until you complete your set.

*Variation for Week 3, Workout 3:* **Banded Tricep Kickbacks**

Get into your tricep kickback position and, holding one resistance band handle in each hand, stand on the resistance band with your feet hip-width apart and perform your tricep kickbacks until you have completed your set. Remember: the wider you stand, the more resistance you will have. If there's too much resistance, bring your feet closer together to decrease it.

*Good things come to those who put in the work.*

# SIX

# Keep It Up— This Is Now Your Lifestyle!

You did it! You conquered twenty-one days of Chi-Keto. I'm so proud of you. This is a gift for yourself and for your future, and all I hope to do is inspire you to keep going with this lifestyle and make it yours. It is possible that at this very moment you don't see a drastic change in the mirror, but I know you *feel* a difference in your energy and in how your clothes fit. So don't give up now. You're just at the tip of the iceberg.

When I began my keto journey a little more than a year ago, I was tapping into my thirties and incredibly aware (because everyone and their *mamá* kept repeating it) that my metabolism was only going to get slower from then on. That didn't sit well with what I was experiencing on the weight front. I mean, I was eating what I considered to be healthy meals, like lentils, and brown rice, and *frijoles de la olla*, and granola in my yogurt . . . but, now that you also know what those foods do to our bodies, we both understand that I wasn't going to get too far with that carb-loaded diet. However, at the time, I was puzzled. I didn't get why, with these "healthy" choices, I still didn't feel good and why the scale was stubbornly refusing to budge. My bloating wasn't going away and my weight wasn't coming off, even though I continuously worked out. I had no idea I was overloading my body with carbs and sugar, spiking up my insulin and basically telling my body to store the excess fat rather than lose it no matter how much exercise I did.

That's when I knew it was time to say goodbye to temporary fixes and really focus on a lifestyle change. I not only hoped to stop suffering through all the yo-yo dieting of my twenties, but also truly yearned to feel better, look better, and have more energy. The last thing I wanted was to actually feel my thirties hitting me hard. I began to come into my own as a woman, and I needed my health and body to reflect this blooming, newfound confidence.

This coincided with another turning point in my life: finally embracing my curves. When I hit thirty, something in me switched. I realized my curves were an asset that I just had to understand better. Since I'm *chaparrita* (a shorty) and curvy, when I gain weight, it spreads evenly throughout my body, so I don't realize it's happening until I see a photo of myself and am like, "Hold up, I look thicker! What happened?" Now that doesn't mean I aspire to be stick thin. When I say we must embrace our curves, I really mean each and every one of us has to press pause, understand our personal body type, and embrace it in all its glory. I know I'm short and I'm never going to have thin and long runway model legs, and that's okay. In my twenties, I was much harder on myself. I felt like I had to look a certain way, but now, in my thirties, I am feeling the self-love. This is who I am, unique and *buenota* just the way I am. All I want now is to improve so I can feel better all around. And I'm getting there.

I no longer live in workout pants; my jeans are actually loose, and it makes my heart skip a beat. This plan really works. Lorenzo didn't realize how much weight I'd lost until he saw an old picture of me the other day. "Wow, wait, I never saw you like that," he exclaimed. Lorenzo has always loved my curves, and loved me for who I am, and loved my legs and butt regardless of my size. So he didn't really notice my gradual change until he saw those photos. And, let me tell you, they shocked me straight too. I suddenly understood what slow and steady really means. I've come a long way and still have a little more to go. Though Lorenzo, who supports me in everything I do, has made one special request: "Whatever you do, you can't lose your booty." It's not going anywhere except up with all of Sarah's booty-toning exercises, so I'm not worried about that.

I've tried to get Lorenzo to join me in my keto-friendly ways, but he's not quite there yet. I'm not going to lie, that still remains a challenge for me. He's not the challenge because he's incredibly supportive, but rather our mealtime as a couple is. When I'm standing in the kitchen making my keto-friendly meal and cooking some frijoles on the side for my partner, that's one of my ultimate challenges. So I turn it into a moment to practice my willpower. And I actually end up getting a kick out of having one of my favorite foods in front of me and choosing not to touch it. It makes me feel so proud. It goes beyond just saying no; this lifestyle is teaching me that I am a strong woman and I have the power to choose, that I got this, that I now have the tools that will continue to help me reinforce my will to lead a healthy life.

My mental clarity and energy are through the roof with Chi-Keto too, and I love it. Before I took off on this journey, I remember having my usual superlong days and not being able to wake up the next morning to work out, or dragging myself out of bed every morning as if starting a new day was pure torture. Now it doesn't even matter if I've gone to sleep at midnight or one in the morning; I will wake up the next day and still get my exercise in. That minor difference has made a huge impact in my life. And because I've been able to work out steadily, my endurance has increased—another change I celebrate every day.

Working out is such a key component in this plan because it not only helps us stay tight and keeps us healthy, it is also the ultimate stress reliever. When I work out with Sarah, sometimes I say, "I need boxing today," because I'm in desperate need of getting rid of some pent-up emotions. If I'm working out on my own, then hopping on my bike does the trick. And, yes, there are days when I just don't want to move, and those are challenging times, but I push myself, and by the end of my workout, I feel like a badass again.

The exercise together with learning how to eat well has truly changed my life. Fueling my body with the right food has helped me endure my many long days and nights of work, like when I was doing *Tengo Talento Mucho Talento* and my workday didn't end until midnight. The keto-friendly meals kept me clearheaded and focused, allowing me to get through the day and night and still have energy to get up and keep going the next day.

I can't believe how far I've come. Looking back to when I started this lifestyle, what I feel most now is relief. The relief of having finally found a way of eating that is healthy and sustainable. The relief of seeing amazing changes that have only helped improve my body and mind, my overall health, and my self-esteem. I've carried my weight issue on my shoulders most of my life, and it became even harder to handle when I began to live my life in the limelight. My weight has always been a thing, a topic of conversation, of gossip, of trolls. So having finally found something that I absolutely love and stand behind 100 percent is also an immense relief.

I'm a huge keto-friendly advocate because I know firsthand how diets feel. I've tried them all, and this is the one I was finally able to stick with way longer than any other one, and I feel the difference. With the bloating and excess weight gone, I've also left behind the baggage of worrying about what other people say or think about my health. Now I know who I am, where I'm going, and why, and no one is going to be able to mess with that. My keto-friendly lifestyle has injected me with a surge of confidence. I feel better, and I don't experience the amount of pressure I used to endure because I know what I'm doing is good for me. This lifestyle has also taught me how to be kind to myself and allow a day in my week to indulge my cravings guilt free.

A few Sundays ago, I went to a Dodgers game and made my two Dodger dogs and a beer my indulgence meal, and I was super happy. There was no guilty little voice filling me with shame with every bite. That has been lifted. I was not worrying about calories or points or net carbs or gaining weight. I was simply enjoying the indulgence knowing that the following day I'd continue with my keto-friendly meals and feel great. We can have our cake and eat it too, and that makes a world of difference.

Vacation time can get a little tricky, but that's when you just have to find your stride and strike a balance that works for you. When Lorenzo and I took off on our honeymoon in Puerto Rico, I would allow myself one indulgence meal a day and remain keto-friendly the rest of the day. So some days I'd keep it keto in the morning and at lunch, and then enjoy a traditional local meal for dinner because I wasn't about to miss out on those *habichuelas* and *mofongo* dishes. However, now that I'm so aware of what I'm putting into my body, I'm not going to lie, at times I was tripping out. I saw the bread and butter on the table, then the *tostones*, then the main dish with a heaping portion of rice, and I knew it was all overflowing with carbs. One night I even said to Lorenzo, "Look, my stomach is flat right now. I'm gonna show you the difference," and when we left the restaurant I looked like I was pregnant . . . um, pregnant with *habichuelas*! He was bloated too! We were rolling out of those restaurants. But we were having fun and enjoying the food and making memories, and I was out of ketosis, but guess what? Doing so didn't reverse all my hard work. I enjoyed the moment and relaxed knowing that once the vacation was over, we'd be home and I'd hop back into my regular keto-friendly way of eating and all would return to my new normal.

The truth is that with any type of diet, if you change the way you eat for the worse you will gain weight. That's why it has to become a lifestyle. By doing that, you will be able to shed any vacation weight gained and get back on track rather than falling down the rabbit hole and reversing all your hard work just because you took a break. Remember, everything in life is about balance.

Now that you've decided to turn this 21-day plan into a lifestyle, what are your new goals? Life is all about short- and long-term goals, and this is no different. I'm a full-fledged woman now. I love who I am, so I simply want to improve what I have, tone up, get healthier, and enhance what I have already learned to embrace. And that's what I hope you will do too. At this point in my journey, I want to continue to work out to give my booty an extra lift and to tone up my arms so I can feel comfortable in sleeveless clothes. I also want my abs to have a little more definition.

My short-term goal weight-wise was aiming to fit comfortably into a size 8, and I'm there now. I can also fit into size 29 pants and, after wearing size large for a long while, I'm down to medium, which fills me with joy. Each time I slide into my everyday jeans and notice they're a little looser around my waist, I celebrate that feeling. Those are the moments when I cheer myself on the most, because each small step is getting me closer to my end goal. And no, it's not a size 0, are you crazy? My long-term goal is to fit into a size 6. Why? Because I was a size 6 about five years ago and I absolutely loved how I felt and looked back then. Plus, I have the cutest little size 6 dress in the back of my closet, and I can't wait to finally put it on again because I so loved how I felt in it and I want to feel that again. It's there, waiting for me like a patient lover, and I know I will be wearing it again soon.

So, yes, like you, I still have work to do, but I'm already so happy. I don't feel as bloated and I don't look as puffy as I used to, and that makes me want to twerk for joy. That carb face is history, and it's such a relief. It's really all in the little things, those small differences that make such an impact in how we feel, and walk, and talk, and carry ourselves.

With Chi-Keto I've been able to expand my food horizons. It may have started as a new way of eating, a new way of losing weight, but it has become so much more. This is not a diet, this is not a journey, this is now my life, and I hope it will be yours too. I want you to be as happy as I am. I hope that after these twenty-one days, the way you are feeling inspires you to keep going with this program. I want you to embrace who you are, I want you to embrace your body. Don't compare your results to anyone else's. Each person is different, so it's important to focus on your own journey and always act based on how *you* feel. Connect with yourself, listen to your body.

As women we feel the difference, we see the difference, we know, so don't let anyone rain on your parade. Celebrate the small accomplishments along the way, even if the only person noticing them is you. Every step is key. And once you start to feel amazing, you won't even care what others think. That's when you'll be ready to turn this into the rest of your life. Because you won't ever want to feel any other way. If you ever feel discouraged or think the differences you are experiencing aren't all that great, remember one thing: the faster you lose weight, the faster you will gain it back. So instead of focusing on how many pounds you're shedding along the way, really make an effort to connect with how you are feeling and everything you are experiencing. Recall the last three weeks: mental clarity came first, then an energy surge, followed by reduced bloating, and that's when the weight began to melt off. Be aware of these stages and celebrate each one along the way. *Al final del día, la vida es para gozarla* (at the end of the day, life is meant to be enjoyed and celebrated). Do it for yourself. You won't regret it.

## WHAT NOW?

Continue using this guide as a cookbook. Look up your favorite recipes and keep them in your weekly rotation. You now also know what a Chi-Keto meal should look like on your plate, with the right amounts of fats, proteins, and carbs. Just remember the basics for your plate: start with a palm-size protein, fill it up with greens and low-carb veggies, add your healthy fats, and you will be all set. When you're on the go, also stick with the basics while eating out. If you're craving a burger, replace the bun with a lettuce wrap, add some cheese and avocado, and call it your satisfaction guarantee. If you are dying for some fajitas, just nix the tortilla and ask for double guacamole or cheese.

And don't slack on your workouts. With Sarah's anywhere/anytime workouts you have no excuses. There's no need for a gym. Just keep her workouts handy on your phone, tablet, or computer by going to bootyfitworkout.com or YouTube.com/bootyfitworkout and follow along if you want to change up your exercise routine. The key to working out is consistency.

Your mind is incredibly powerful. What you give attention to will have power over you. So stay focused on your goals and don't let anything distract you. Always remember, you are a *chingona* and you got this!

Nothing can dim your light.
Shine on, Chi-Keto queen!
#BeeKind
#BeeStrong
#BeeYou

# Acknowledgments

**FROM CHIQUIS:**

I want to thank my mama for being the biggest influence in every aspect of my life. The epitome of a *chingona* who taught me to go after whatever I want and to embrace my God-given body while always leaving room to strive for more.

To YOU, the boss bee who loves herself enough to have picked up this book and made the decision to become a better version of herself. You're a *chingona*! I dedicate this book to you and am so grateful to be a part of your journey.

**FROM SARAH:**

To my beautiful mom: I am so grateful for you and all that you have instilled in me about working hard, never giving up, and always doing things with integrity. I love you.

Jaime: Thank you for your constant support, love, and being the best teammate I could ask for. *Te amo.*

Lala, Aaron, Claudia, Realiz, Nikki, Amy, Suzy, Tasha, Bri, Yoli, and Lilo: Thank you for your unconditional love and support throughout this journey. I am so grateful for each and every one of you. Tequila on me!

To Cecilia: Thank you for your patience, kindness, and for putting this vision into words.

To Johanna, Michelle, Melanie, and Atria/Simon and Schuster: Thank you for believing in this project and making all of this possible. It definitely takes a village.

# Index

## A

A la Chi-Taco Salad, 82–83
*adobo*, 127
*Aguacate Relleno*, 57
*Aguachile*, 79–80
alcoholic beverages
  beer, 146
  on Chi-Keto diet, 26, 109,
    141–42
  recipes, 141–46
alternating bicep curls
    (exercises), 46, 164
alternating lunges (exercise),
    40, 166
alternating shoulder presses
    (exercise), 41, 168
*arroz con frijoles*, 6
*arroz con leche*, 21, 156
*arroz rojo*, 113
Arugula Salad, 117, 138
Atkins diet, 5
Avocado Crema, 61
avocado recipes
  *Aguacate Relleno*, 57
  Avocado Crema, 61
  Bacon Avocado Bomb, 67
  Bacon Guacamole Chicken
    Bomb, 105–6
  Baked Avocado with Bacon
    and Cheese, 57

Chi-Muffins, 58
Chicken Taco Salad with
    Chipotle Ranch Dressing,
    82–83
Chocolate Green Creamy
    Smoothie, 75
Ground Turkey Stuffed
    Avocados, 93
Guacamole, 106
Pumpkin Spice Coffee
    Smoothies, 74
Sausage Torta, 69
*Ay Mojito, Qué Rico*, 143

## B

back rows (exercise), 34,
    166–67
Bacon Avocado Bomb, 67
Bacon Guacamole Chicken
    Bomb, 105–6
bacon recipes
  Bacon Avocado Bomb, 67
  Bacon Guacamole Chicken
    Bomb, 105–6
  Bacon-Wrapped Jalapeño
    Poppers, 152
  Baked Avocado with Bacon
    and Cheese, 57
  Tuna Bacon Salad,
    103

Bacon-Wrapped Jalapeño
    Poppers, 152
Baked Avocado with Bacon and
    Cheese, 57
banded bicep curls
    (exercise), 34, 164
banded glute bridges
    (exercise), 40, 163
banded glute kickbacks
    (exercise), 41, 47,
    169
banded squats (exercise), 34,
    164
banded tricep dips
    (exercises), 47, 169
beans (*frijoles*), 6, 19, 21, 22,
    154
beer, 146
Berries and Cream, 159
beverages
  alcoholic, 26, 109, 141–46
  craving sweet drinks, 77
  sparkling water, 77
  sweeteners in, 20
  water, 14, 20, 27
bingeing, 18
Blueberry Cheesecake Bars,
    63
Blueberry Chia Pudding,
    68

breakfast
about, 51
menu plans, 31–32, 37–38, 43–44
breakfast recipes, 53–75
*Aguacate Relleno*, 57
Bacon Avocado Bomb, 67
Baked Avocado with Bacon and Cheese, 57
Blueberry Cheesecake Bars, 63
Blueberry Chia Pudding, 68
Cheesy Turkey Egg Tacos, 72
Chi-Keto Horchata Smoothie, 60
Chi-Keto Pancakes, 70
Chi-Muffins, 58
*Chilaquiles con Chicharrón* and Avocado Crema, 61
Chocolate Blueberry Pancakes, 62
Chocolate Green Creamy Smoothie, 75
Chorizo Breakfast Bowl, 56
Coconut Pancakes, 65
Crispy Cinnamon Almond Waffles, 73
Dried Beef with Eggs, 64
Eggs with Tomato Sauce, 53–55
Fajita Frittata, 59
Ham and Cheese Omelet Stuffed in Bell Pepper, 66
*Huevos Rancheros*, 53–55
*Machaca con Huevos*, 64
Portobello Egg Toast, 71
Pumpkin Spice Coffee Smoothies, 74
Sausage Torta, 69
Tex-Mex Avocado Ham Eggs, 58
breaking habits, 19
Broiled Salmon with Arugula Salad, 138

burger recipes
Chi-Keto Burgers, 85
keto substitute for buns, 21
Portobello Bun Turkey Cheeseburger with Pico de Gallo, 85
Protein-Style Parmesan Cheese Chicken Burger Verde, 84
Spicy Mozzarella Chicken Burger Ranch Salad, 100

C

*café con leche*, 51
*Camarones a la Diabla* with Mexican Kale Salad, 132–33
carbs
in Atkins diet, 5
beans (*frijoles*), 6, 19, 21, 22, 154
fruits, 6, 7, 8
good/bad carbs (list), 7–8
in keto diet, 1, 2, 6–8, 9
ketosis, 1–2
Latino foods, 6
low-carb foods, 6
lowering, 1
net carbs, 7
portion size, 12–13
quantity allowed, 6
sugar alcohols, 6
*Carne a la Tampiqueña* with Roasted Zucchini, 129–30
*Carne Asada* with Chimichurri in Lettuce Wraps, 125–26
Carnitas with Jalapeño Poppers, 86–87
cauliflower, store-bought products, 49

Cauliflower Chorizo over Chicharrón Nachos, 115
Cauliflower Elote, 149
cauliflower recipes
Cauliflower Chorizo over Chicharrón Nachos, 115
Cauliflower Elote, 149
Cauliflower Rice, 113
Chicken Fajitas with Mexican Cauliflower Rice, 113–14
*Fajitas a la Flor*, 113–14
Fried Chicken with Mashed Garlic Cauliflower, 120–21
"Nacho-Bitch," 115
Prosciutto Arugula Pizza, 91–92
Cauliflower Rice, 113
"cheat meal," 17
cheese recipes
Bacon-Wrapped Jalapeño Poppers, 152
Baked Avocado with Bacon and Cheese, 57
Blueberry Cheesecake Bars, 63
Cauliflower Chorizo over Chicharrón Nachos, 115
Cauliflower Elote, 149
Cheesy Turkey Egg Tacos, 72
Chicken-and-Cheese-Stuffed Poblano Peppers, 81
Chicken Breast in Cheese and Spinach Sauce, 97
Chicken Cheese Quesadilla, 99
Chicken Enchilada Bowl, 124
Chicken Sausage Vegetable Skillet, 123
Chicken Taquitos, 137
Chicken Tortilla Soup, 90
Chili for the Soul, 139

Creamy Chicken Tomato
      Noodles, 122
Cucumber and Cheese Salad,
      131
Ham and Cheese Omelet
      Stuffed in Bell Pepper, 6
Ham and Cheesy Egg
      Rollup, 151
Keto Refried Beans, 154
Lemon Arugula Parmesan
      Salad, 117
Mozzarella Tostadas, 80
"Nacho-Bitch," 115
Portobello Bun Turkey
      Cheeseburger with Pico
      de Gallo, 85
Protein-Style Parmesan
      Cheese Chicken Burger
      Verde, 84
Spicy Mozzarella Chicken
      Burger Ranch Salad, 100
tostadas, 21, 80, 116
Turkey-Wrapped
      Mozzarella Sticks, 153
Cheesy Turkey Egg Tacos, 72
chest presses (exercise), 46
Chi-Keto Burgers, 85
Chi-Keto diet, xv, xvi, 171–76
      advantages of, 172–73
      alcoholic beverages, 26, 109,
            141–46
      bingeing, 18
      birth of, xv
      carbs in, 6–8
      Chingona Tips, 6, 14, 18, 21,
            27, 29, 30, 36, 42, 44, 51,
            77, 109, 147, 163
      cravings, 18, 21, 63
      drinking water, 14, 20, 27
      exercising. See exercises;
            workout plan
      falling off the wagon, 22
      fats in, 3–5, 9, 14
      feeling good, 15–16

getting back on track, 22–23,
      25
goals for, 25–26
Happy Hour, 26, 31n, 37n,
      143–46
indulgence day, 6, 17, 18,
      22, 174
keto flu, 19–20
keto-friendly fruits (list), 8
loving yourself, 23–24
meal schedule, 29
motivation, 42
overall health, 15–16
pantry items, 27–28
portion size, 12–13
proteins in, 4–5, 14
recipes. See recipes
roadblocks at first, 19–22
self–image and, 23–24
self-sabotage, 22, 23
snacks, 13, 14, 25, 26, 29,
      30, 31, 43, 49, 147–59
"sweet tooth," 30, 43, 63,
      147
sweeteners, 8
temptation and, 20–21
typical plate, 13
vacations and, 174
weighing yourself, 14–15
weight loss and, 175
See also 21-day plan; workout
      plan
Chi-Keto Friendly Tortillas,
      54, 99
Chi-Keto Horchata Smoothie,
      60
Chi-Keto Pancakes, 70
Chi-Keto Tacos, 111–12
Chi-Muffins, 58
chia seed recipes
      Arroz con Leche, 156
      Blueberry Chia Pudding, 68
Chicken-and-Cheese-Stuffed
      Poblano Peppers, 81

Chicken Breast in Cheese and
      Spinach Sauce, 97
Chicken Cheese Quesadilla, 99
Chicken Chipotle Casserole, 94
Chicken Enchilada Bowl, 124
Chicken Fajitas with
      Mexican Cauliflower
      Rice, 113–14
Chicken Sausage Vegetable
      Skillet, 123
Chicken Taco Salad with
      Chipotle Ranch
      Dressing, 82–83
Chicken Taquitos, 137
Chicken Tortilla Soup, 90
Chilaquiles con Chicharrón and
      Avocado Crema, 61
Chile Gordo, 81
Chile Relleno with Ground
      Chicken, 98
chiles, 28
Chili for the Soul, 139
Chimichurri, 126
Chingona Tips, 6, 14, 18, 21,
      27, 29, 30, 36, 42, 44, 51,
      77, 109, 147, 163
Chipotle Ranch Dressing,
      82–83
chocolate-covered strawberries,
      158
chocolate recipes
      Chocolate Blueberry
            Pancakes, 62
      Chocolate Green Creamy
            Smoothie, 75
      Chocolate Strawberry
            Mousse, 158
      Mexican Hot Chocolate
            Pudding, 157
Chorizo Breakfast Bowl, 56
Cilantro Crema, 61, 111
Cilantro Lime Dressing, 89
Coconut Chicken Tenders, 136
Coconut Pancakes, 65

coffee, 51
  Pumpkin Spice Coffee
    Smoothies, 74
*Costillas de Puerco en Adobo*
    *con Ensalada de Nopales*,
    127–28
cravings, 18, 21, 63
Creamy Chicken Tomato
    Noodles, 122
*crema* recipes
  Avocado Crema, 61
  Cilantro Crema, 61, 111
Crispy Cinnamon Almond
    Waffles, 73
crunches (exercise), 34, 40, 46,
    167
Cucumber and Cheese Salad,
    131

**D**

dairy foods, shopping lists, 31,
    38, 44
dessert recipes
  Berries and Cream, 159
  Blueberry Chia Pudding, 68
  Chia Seed *Arroz con Leche*,
    156
  Fruit Cup with Tajín, 155
  Mexican Hot Chocolate
    Pudding, 157
diets
  Atkins diet, 5
  failure of, xii, 11, 12, 17
  multitasking and, 11
  starving yourself, 14
  *See also* Chi-Keto diet; foods
dinner
  about, 109
  menu plans, 31–32, 37–38,
    43–44
Dried Beef with Eggs, 64
drinking water, 14, 20, 27
dumbbell bicep curls
    (exercise), 40, 164

dumbbell squats (exercise), 40,
    165

**E**

*Eat Fat, Get Thin* (Hyman), 3
egg recipes
  Cheesy Turkey Egg Tacos, 72
  Chi-Keto Friendly Tortillas,
    54, 99
  Chi-Keto Pancakes, 70
  Chi-Muffins, 58
  Chorizo Breakfast Bowl, 56
  Dried Beef with Eggs, 64
  Eggs with Tomato Sauce,
    53–55
  Fajita Frittata, 59
  Ham and Cheese Omelet
    Stuffed in Bell Pepper, 66
  Ham and Cheesy Egg Rollup,
    151
  Portobello Egg Toast, 71
  Sausage Torta, 69
  Tex-Mex Avocado Ham Eggs,
    58
Eggs with Tomato Sauce, 53–55
electrolytes, replenishing, 20
*elote*
  Cauliflower Elote, 149
  keto substitute for, 21, 149
*enchiladas*, 94
  Chicken Enchilada Bowl, 124
*Ensalada de Nopales*, 127–28
exercises, 16–17, 27, 161–69
  alternating bicep curls, 46,
    164
  alternating lunges, 40, 166
  alternating shoulder presses,
    41, 168
  back rows, 34, 166–67
  banded bicep curls, 34,
    164
  banded glute bridges, 40, 163
  banded glute kickbacks, 41,
    47, 169

banded squats, 34, 164
banded tricep dips, 47,
    169
chest presses, 46
crunches, 34, 40, 46, 167
dumbbell bicep curls, 40,
    164
dumbbell squats, 40, 165
glute bridges, 34, 46, 163
glute bridges to chest
    presses, 46, 163–64
glute kickbacks, 35, 168
modified push-ups, 40
mountain climbers, 35, 41,
    47, 168
plank, 34, 40, 46, 165
plank rows, 46, 167
push-ups, 46, 166
shoulder presses, 35, 168
single-arm back rows, 40,
    167
skipping a workout, 163
squats to shoulder presses,
    46, 47, 165, 168
stagnant lunges, 34, 165
stagnant lunges to bicep
    curls, 46, 166
tips for, 161–63
tricep dips, 35, 41, 169
warm-up, 162
*See also* workout plan

**F**

Fajita Frittata, 59
*fajita* recipes
  Chicken Fajitas with
    Mexican Cauliflower
    Rice, 113–14
  Fajita Frittata, 59
  *Fajitas a la Flor*, 113–14
  Steak Fajita Rolls, 104
  Steak Fajita Salad with Cilantro
    Lime Dressing, 88–89
*Fajitas a la Flor*, 113–14

falling off the wagon, 22
fats
  good/bad fats (list), 4
  healthy fats, 3
  hydrogenated and partially
    hydrogenated, 3
  in keto diet, 2–3, 9, 14
  low-fat craze, 2–3
  monounsaturated and
    polyunsaturated, 3
  portion size, 13
  saturated fats, 3
  trans fats, 3
*Filete de Pescado* with Cucumber
    and Cheese Salad, 131
fish and seafood recipes
  *Aguachile*, 79–80
  Broiled Salmon with Arugula
    Salad, 138
  *Camarones a la Diabla* with
    Mexican Kale Salad,
    132–33
  *Filete de Pescado* with
    Cucumber and Cheese
    Salad, 131
  Roasted Salmon with Lime
    Cream Sauce and
    Asparagus, 118–19
  Shrimp Ceviche with Keto
    Tostada, 116
  Shrimp Stir-Fry, 107
  Tuna Bacon Salad, 103
foods
  beans (*frijoles*), 6, 19, 21, 22,
    154
  best foods for, 27
  beverages, 20
  fruits, 6, 7, 8, 13
  good/bad carbs (list), 7–8
  good/bad fats (list), 4
  good/bad proteins (list), 5
  good fruits (list), 8
  good vegetables (list), 7
  keto-friendly fruits (list), 8

Latino foods, xv, xvi, 6
  low-carb foods, 6
  meal schedule, 29
  pantry items, 27–28
  portion size, 12–13
  processed meats, 5
  shopping lists, 32–33, 38–39,
    44–45
  snacks, 13, 14, 25, 26, 29,
    30, 31, 43, 49, 147–59
  typical Chi-Keto plate, 13
  *See also* meals; recipes
Fried Chicken with Mashed
    Garlic Cauliflower,
    120–21
*frijoles*, 6, 19, 21, 22, 154
Fruit Cup with Tajín, 155
fruit juice, 77
fruit recipes
  Berries and Cream, 159
  Blueberry Cheesecake Bars, 63
  Blueberry Chia Pudding, 68
  Chocolate Blueberry
    Pancakes, 62
  Chocolate Strawberry
    Mousse, 158
  Fruit Cup with Tajín, 155
fruits, 6, 7, 8
  keto-friendly fruits (list), 8
  shopping lists, 31–32, 38–39,
    44–45
  as snack, 13

G
getting back on track, 22–23
glute bridges (exercise), 34, 46,
    163
glute bridges to chest presses
    (exercise), 46, 163–64
glute kickbacks (exercise), 35,
    168
Grilled Chicken with Lemon
    Arugula Parmesan Salad,
    117

Ground Turkey Stuffed
    Avocados, 93
Guacamole, 106

H
habits, 19
Ham and Cheese Omelet
    Stuffed in Bell Pepper, 66
Ham and Cheesy Egg Rollup,
    151
Happy Hour
  about, 26, 31*n*, 37*n*, 141–42
  recipes, 143–46
healthy fats, 3
horchata, Chi-Keto Horchata
    Smoothie, 60
*Huevos Rancheros*, 53–55
hydration, 20, 27
hydrogenated fats, 3
Hyman, Mark, 3

I
indulgence day, 16, 17, 18, 22,
    174
insomnia, keto flu and, 19, 20
irritability, keto flu and, 19, 20

J
Jalapeño Poppers, 87

K
keto diet (ketogenic diet)
  basics of, 1–9
  calculating numbers
    (macronutrients), 12–13
  carbs in, 1, 2, 6–8, 9
  early efforts at, xii–xiv
  fats in, 2–3, 4, 9, 14
  healthy fats, 3
  ketosis, 1–2
  for Latino-food lovers,
    xv, xvi, 6
  macronutrients, 2, 5
  principle of, 1

keto diet (*cont.*)
  protein in, 2, 5, 9, 14
  recipes. *See* recipes
  *See also* Chi-Keto diet; foods;
    21-day plan
keto flu, 19–20
Keto Refried Beans, 154
ketosis, 1–2
Koudouzian, Sarah, xiii–xv, 11,
  14, 23, 25, 144

L

lactose intolerance, 3–4
Latino foods, xv, xvi, 6
  *adobo*, 127
  *arroz and frijoles*, 6
  *arroz con leche*, 21, 156
  *arroz rojo*, 113
  *café con leche*, 51
  *chilaquiles*, 61
  *chile relleno*, 98
  *elote*, 21, 149
  *enchiladas*, 94, 124
  *fajitas*, 59, 88–89, 104
  *frijoles*, 6, 19, 21, 22, 154
  horchata, 60
  *huevos rancheros*, 53–55
  indulging in on keto, 6, 17,
    18, 22
  *machaca*, 64
  mojitos, 143
  *mole*, 95–96
  nachos, 115
  nopales, 95–96, 127–28
  *plátanos*, 6
  *quesadillas*, 99
  substitutes for, 21, 36
  *tacos*, 72, 111–12, 137
  as temptation, 21–22
  tequila, 144, 145
  *tortillas*, 6, 21, 36, 54, 99
  *tostadas*, 21, 80, 116
Lemon Arugula Parmesan
  Salad, 117

Lemon Pepper Chicken Wings
  with Ranch Dressing, 135
Lettuce-Wrapped Chicken
  Tacos with Cilantro
  Crema, 111–12
Lime Cream Sauce, 118
low-fat craze, 2–3
lunch
  about, 77
  menu plans, 31–32, 37–38,
    43–44

M

*Machaca con Huevos*, 64
macronutrients, 2, 5, 11–12, 13
meals
  breakfast, 51
  dinner, 109
  lunch, 77
  sample menus, 31–32,
    37–38, 43–44
  schedule for, 29
  *See also* foods; recipes
meat, shopping lists, 32, 39, 45
meat recipes
  A la Chi-Taco Salad, 82–83
  Bacon Avocado Bomb, 67
  Bacon Guacamole Chicken
    Bomb, 105–6
  Bacon-Wrapped Jalapeño
    Poppers, 152
  Baked Avocado with Bacon
    and Cheese, 57
  *Carne a la Tampiqueña*
    with Roasted Zucchini,
    129–30
  *Carne Asada* with Chimichurri
    in Lettuce Wraps, 125–26
  Carnitas with Jalapeño
    Poppers, 86–87
  Cauliflower Chorizo over
    Chicharrón Nachos, 115
  Cheesy Turkey Egg Tacos, 72
  Chi-Keto Burgers, 85

Chi-Keto Tacos, 111–12
Chicken-and-Cheese-Stuffed
  Poblano Peppers, 81
Chicken Breast in Cheese
  and Spinach Sauce, 97
Chicken Cheese Quesadilla, 99
Chicken Chipotle Casserole,
  94
Chicken Enchilada Bowl, 124
Chicken Fajitas with Mexican
  Cauliflower Rice, 113–14
Chicken Sausage Vegetable
  Skillet, 123
Chicken Taco Salad with
  Chipotle Ranch Dressing,
  82–83
Chicken Taquitos, 137
Chicken Tortilla Soup, 90
*Chile Relleno* with Ground
  Chicken, 98
Chili for the Soul, 139
Coconut Chicken Tenders, 136
*Costillas de Puerco en Adobo
  con Ensalada de Nopales*,
  127–28
Creamy Chicken Tomato
  Noodles, 122
Dried Beef with Eggs, 64
*Fajitas a la Flor*, 113–14
Fried Chicken with Mashed
  Garlic Cauliflower,
  120–21
Grilled Chicken with Lemon
  Arugula Parmesan Salad,
  117
Ground Turkey Stuffed
  Avocados, 93
Ham and Cheesy Egg Rollup,
  151
Lemon Pepper Chicken Wings
  with Ranch Dressing, 135
Lettuce-Wrapped Chicken
  Tacos with Cilantro
  Crema, 111–12

Mexican Meatsa, 134
Mexican Pulled Pork with Stuffed Peppers, 86–87
"Nacho-Bitch," 115
Not Your Basic Chick, 84
*Pechuga de Pollo en Salsa de Queso y Espinaca*, 97
*Pollo a la Plancha*, 117
*Pollo en Mole Verde* with Hemp Seed Rice, 95–96
Portobello Bun Turkey Cheeseburger with Pico de Gallo, 85
Prosciutto Arugula Pizza, 91–92
Protein-Style Parmesan Cheese Chicken Burger Verde, 84
Sausage Torta, 69
Spicy Mozzarella Chicken Burger Ranch Salad, 100
Steak Fajita Rolls, 104
Steak Fajita Salad with Cilantro Lime Dressing, 88–89
Stuffed Zucchini Boats, 102
Tuna Bacon Salad, 103
Turkey-Wrapped Mozzarella Sticks, 153
menu plans
Week 1, 31–32
Week 2, 37–38
Week 3, 43–44
Mexican Hot Chocolate Pudding, 157
Mexican Kale Salad, 132–33
Mexican Meatsa, 134
Mexican Pulled Pork with Stuffed Peppers, 86–87
*Michelada*, 146
milk, keto substitute for, 21, 51
modified push-ups (exercises), 40
Mojitos, 143
*mole*, 95–96
monounsaturated fats, 3

motivation, 42
mountain climbers (exercise), 35, 41, 47, 168
Mozzarella Tostadas, 80

N
"Nacho-Bitch," 115
net carbs, calculating, 7
nopales
*Ensalada de Nopales*, 127–28
*Pollo en Mole Verde* with Hemp Seed Rice, 95–96
Not Your Basic Chick, 84
nuts
*Pepinos Locos*, 150
as snack, 14, 147

O
oils and vinegars, 28

P
*Paloma Blanca*, 145
pancakes and waffles
Chi-Keto Pancakes, 70
Chocolate Blueberry Pancakes, 62
Coconut Pancakes, 65
Crispy Cinnamon Almond Waffles, 73
pantry items, 27–28
partially hydrogenated fats, 3
pasta, zoodles, 21, 49, 122
*Pechuga de Pollo en Salsa de Queso y Espinaca*, 97
*Pepinos Locos*, 150
peppers and chiles
Bacon-Wrapped Jalapeño Poppers, 152
Carnitas with Jalapeño Poppers, 86–87
Chicken-and-Cheese-Stuffed Poblano Peppers, 81
Chicken Chipotle Casserole, 94

*Chile Gordo*, 81
*Chile Relleno* with Ground Chicken, 98
Ham and Cheese Omelet Stuffed in Bell Pepper, 66
Jalapeño Poppers, 87
Mexican Pulled Pork with Stuffed Peppers, 86–87
Steak Fajita Rolls, 104
Tomatillo-Pasilla Sauce, 93
Pesto, 92
pizza recipes
Mexican Meatsa, 134
Prosciutto Arugula Pizza, 91–92
plank (exercise), 34, 40, 46, 165
plank rows (exercise), 46, 167
*plátanos*, 6
*Pollo a la Plancha*, 117
*Pollo en Mole Verde* with Hemp Seed Rice, 95–96
polyunsaturated fats, 3
poppers, Bacon-Wrapped Jalapeño Poppers, 152
portion size, 12–13
Portobello Bun Turkey Cheeseburger with Pico de Gallo, 85
Portobello Egg Toast, 71
processed meats, 5
produce. *See* fruits; vegetables
Prosciutto Arugula Pizza, 91–92
protein
good/bad proteins (list), 5
in keto diet, 2, 5, 9, 14
moderation in keto diet, 5
portion size, 5, 14
processed meats, 5
Protein-Style Parmesan Cheese Chicken Burger Verde, 84

proteins, shopping lists, 32, 39, 45
pudding recipes
    Blueberry Chia Pudding, 68
    Mexican Hot Chocolate Pudding, 157
Pumpkin Spice Coffee Smoothies, 74
push-ups (exercise), 46, 166

## Q

*quesadillas*, 99

## R

Ranch Dressing, 101, 135
recipes, xv–xvi, 25, 49–159
    A la Chi-Taco Salad, 82–83
    *Adobo*, 127
    *Aguacate Relleno*, 57
    *Aguachile*, 79–80
    alcoholic beverages, 143–46
    Arugula Salad, 117, 138
    *Ay Mojito, Qué Rico*, 143
    Bacon Avocado Bomb, 67
    Bacon Guacamole Chicken Bomb, 105–6
    Bacon-Wrapped Jalapeño Poppers, 152
    Baked Avocado with Bacon and Cheese, 57
    Berries and Cream, 159
    Blueberry Cheesecake Bars, 63
    Blueberry Chia Pudding, 68
    Broiled Salmon with Arugula Salad, 138
    *Camarones a la Diabla* with Mexican Kale Salad, 132–33
    *Carne a la Tampiqueña* with Roasted Zucchini, 129–30
    *Carne Asada* with Chimichurri in Lettuce Wraps, 125–26

Carnitas with Jalapeño Poppers, 86–87
Cauliflower Chorizo over Chicharrón Nachos, 115
Cauliflower Elote, 149
Cauliflower Rice, 113
Cheesy Turkey Egg Tacos, 72
Chi-Keto Burgers, 85
Chi-Keto Friendly Tortillas, 54, 99
Chi-Keto Horchata Smoothie, 60
Chi-Keto Pancakes, 70
Chi-Keto Tacos, 111–12
Chi-Muffins, 58
Chia Seed *Arroz con Leche*, 156
Chicken-and-Cheese-Stuffed Poblano Peppers, 81
Chicken Breast in Cheese and Spinach Sauce, 97
Chicken Cheese Quesadilla, 99
Chicken Chipotle Casserole, 94
Chicken Enchilada Bowl, 124
Chicken Fajitas with Mexican Cauliflower Rice, 113–14
Chicken Sausage Vegetable Skillet, 123
Chicken Taco Salad with Chipotle Ranch Dressing, 82–83
Chicken Taquitos, 137
Chicken Tortilla Soup, 90
*Chilaquiles con Chicharrón* and Avocado Crema, 61
*Chile Gordo*, 81
*Chile Relleno* with Ground Chicken, 98
Chili for the Soul, 139
Chimichurri, 126
Chipotle Ranch Dressing, 82–83
Chocolate Blueberry Pancakes, 62

Chocolate Green Creamy Smoothie, 75
Chocolate Strawberry Mousse, 158
Chorizo Breakfast Bowl, 56
Cilantro Crema, 61, 111
Cilantro Lime Dressing, 89
Coconut Chicken Tenders, 136
Coconut Pancakes, 65
*Costillas de Puerco en Adobo con Ensalada de Nopales*, 127–28
Creamy Chicken Tomato Noodles, 122
Crispy Cinnamon Almond Waffles, 73
Cucumber and Cheese Salad, 131
Dried Beef with Eggs, 64
Eggs with Tomato Sauce, 53–55
*Ensalada de Nopales*, 127–28
Fajita Frittata, 59
*Fajitas a la Flor*, 113–14
*Filete de Pescado* with Cucumber and Cheese Salad, 131
Fried Chicken with Mashed Garlic Cauliflower, 120–21
Fruit Cup with Tajín, 155
Grilled Chicken with Lemon Arugula Parmesan Salad, 117
Ground Turkey Stuffed Avocados, 93
Guacamole, 106
Ham and Cheese Omelet Stuffed in Bell Pepper, 66
Ham and Cheesy Egg Rollup, 151

Happy Hour recipes, 143–46
*Huevos Rancheros*, 53–55
Jalapeño Poppers, 87
Keto Refried Beans, 154
Lemon Pepper Chicken Wings with Ranch Dressing, 135
Lettuce-Wrapped Chicken Tacos with Cilantro Crema, 111–12
Lime Cream Sauce, 118
*Machaca con Huevos*, 64
Mexican Hot Chocolate Pudding, 157
Mexican Kale Salad, 132–33
Mexican Meatsa, 134
Mexican Pulled Pork with Stuffed Peppers, 86–87
*Michelada*, 146
Mozzarella Tostadas, 80
"Nacho-Bitch," 115
Not Your Basic Chick, 84
*Paloma Blanca*, 145
*Pechuga de Pollo en Salsa de Queso y Espinaca*, 97
*Pepinos Locos*, 150
Pesto, 92
*Pollo a la Plancha*, 117
*Pollo en Mole Verde* with Hemp Seed Rice, 95–96
Portobello Bun Turkey Cheeseburger with Pico de Gallo, 85
Portobello Egg Toast, 71
Prosciutto Arugula Pizza, 91–92
Protein-Style Parmesan Cheese Chicken Burger Verde, 84
Pumpkin Spice Coffee Smoothies, 74
Ranch Dressing, 101, 135

Roasted Salmon with Lime Cream Sauce and Asparagus, 118–19
Sausage Torta, 69
Shrimp Ceviche with Keto Tostada, 116
Shrimp Stir-Fry, 107
Spicy Mozzarella Chicken Burger Ranch Salad, 100
Spinach Sauce, 97
Steak Fajita Rolls, 104
Steak Fajita Salad with Cilantro Lime Dressing, 88–89
Stuffed Zucchini Boats, 102
*Te Amo Tequila*, 144
Tex-Mex Avocado Ham Eggs, 58
Tomatillo-Pasilla Sauce, 93
Tomato Sauce, 55
Tuna Bacon Salad, 103
Turkey-Wrapped Mozzarella Sticks, 153
rice, keto substitute for, 21, 113
Roasted Salmon with Lime Cream Sauce and Asparagus, 118–19

**S**

salad dressings
Chipotle Ranch Dressing, 82–83
Cilantro Lime Dressing, 89
Ranch Dressing, 101, 135
salad recipes
A la Chi-Taco Salad, 82–83
Arugula Salad, 117, 138
Chicken Taco Salad with Chipotle Ranch Dressing, 82–83
Cucumber and Cheese Salad, 131
*Ensalada de Nopales*, 127–28

Lemon Arugula Parmesan Salad, 117
Mexican Kale Salad, 132–33
Spicy Mozzarella Chicken Burger Ranch Salad, 100
Steak Fajita Salad with Cilantro Lime Dressing, 88–89
Tuna Bacon Salad, 103
saturated fats, 3
sauce recipes
*Adobo*, 127
Chimichurri, 126
Lime Cream Sauce, 118
Spinach Sauce, 97
Tomatillo-Pasilla Sauce, 93
Tomato Sauce, 55
Sausage Torta, 69
seafood
shopping lists, 32, 39, 45
*See also* fish and seafood recipes
self–image, 23–24
self-sabotage, 22, 23
shopping, when hungry, 44
shopping list
for dairy foods, 31, 38, 44
for Happy Hour, 141
for proteins, 32, 39, 45
for snacks, 148
Week 1, 32–33
Week 2, 38–39
Week 3, 44–45
shoulder presses (exercise), 35, 168
Shrimp Ceviche with Keto Tostada, 116
single-arm back rows (exercise), 40, 167
sleep, keto flu and, 20
smoothies
Chi-Keto Horchata Smoothie, 60
Chocolate Green Creamy Smoothie, 75

smoothies (*cont.*)
  Pumpkin Spice Coffee
    Smoothies, 74
snack recipes, 149–59
  Bacon-Wrapped Jalapeño
    Poppers, 152
  Berries and Cream, 159
  Cauliflower Elote, 149
  Chia Seed *Arroz con Leche*,
    156
  Chocolate Strawberry
    Mousse, 158
  Fruit Cup with Tajín, 155
  Ham and Cheesy Egg Rollup,
    151
  Keto Refried Beans, 154
  Mexican Hot Chocolate Pud-
    ding, 157
  *Pepinos Locos*, 150
  Turkey-Wrapped Mozzarella
    Sticks, 153
snacks, 13, 14, 25, 26, 29, 30,
    31, 43, 49, 147–59
soda, 77
soup recipe. *See* Chicken Tortilla
    Soup
sparkling water, 77
spices and seasonings, 27–28
Spicy Mozzarella Chicken
    Burger Ranch Salad, 100
Spinach Sauce, 97
squats to shoulder presses
    (exercise), 46, 47, 165,
    168
stagnant lunges (exercise), 34,
    165
stagnant lunges to bicep curls
    (exercise), 46, 166
starving yourself, 14
Steak Fajita Rolls, 104
Steak Fajita Salad with Cilantro
    Lime Dressing, 88–89
stir fry recipes, Shrimp Stir-Fry,
    107

Stuffed Zucchini Boats, 102
sugar, avoiding, 7, 8
sugar alcohols, 6, 8
"sweet tooth," 30, 43, 63, 147
sweeteners, 8, 20, 51

**T**
taco recipes
  A la Chi-Taco Salad, 82–83
  Cheesy Turkey Egg Tacos, 72
  Chi-Keto Tacos, 111–12
  Chicken Taquitos, 137
  Lettuce-Wrapped Chicken
    Tacos with Cilantro
    Crema, 111–12
*Te Amo Tequila*, 144
temptation, 20–21
tequila, 144, 145
Tex-Mex Avocado Ham Eggs,
    58
Tomatillo-Pasilla Sauce,
    93
Tomato Sauce, 55
*tortillas*, 6, 36
  Chi-Keto Friendly Tortillas,
    54, 99
  keto substitute for, 21
*tostadas*
  keto substitute for, 21, 80
  Shrimp Ceviche with Keto
    Tostada, 116
trans fats, 3
tricep dips (exercise), 35, 41,
    169
Tuna Bacon Salad, 103
Turkey-Wrapped Mozzarella
    Sticks, 153
21-day plan, xvi, 25–47
  breakfast, 51
  breakfast recipes, 53–75
  pantry items, 27–28
  prepping for, 25–28
  Week 1, 30–35
    menu, 31–32

    shopping list, 32–33
    workout, 34–35
  Week 2, 36–41
    menu, 37–38
    shopping list, 38–39
    workout, 40–41
  Week 3, 42–47
    menu, 43–44
    shopping list, 44–45
    workout, 46–47
  *See also* Chi-Keto diet;
    recipes

**V**
vacations, 174
vegetables
  good vegetables (list), 7–8
  portion size, 12–13
  shopping lists, 31–32, 38–39,
    44–45

**W**
water, 14, 20, 27
Week 1, 30
  menu plan, 31–32
  shopping list, 32–33
  workout plan, 34–35
Week 2, 36
  menu plan, 37–38
  shopping list, 38–39
  workout plan, 40–41
Week 3, 42
  menu plan, 43–44
  shopping list, 44–45
  workout plan, 46–47
weighing yourself, 14–15
willpower, 21
wine, 109
workout plan, 16–17, 161–62
  before you start, 162–63
  playlists for, 34, 40, 46
  skipping a workout, 163
  warm-up, 162
  Week 1, 34–35

Week 2, 40–41
Week 3, 46–47
*See also* exercises

Z

zoodles, 21, 49, 122
zucchini recipes
   *Carne a la Tampiqueña*
      with Roasted Zucchini,
      129–30
   Creamy Chicken Tomato
      Noodles, 122
   Stuffed Zucchini Boats, 102
   zoodles, 21, 49, 122

JANNEY MARÍN RIVERA—better known as Chiquis—is an artist, entrepreneur, philanthropist, and television personality. She first captivated her audience on reality shows with her late mom, Jenni Rivera, and their family. She now stars alongside her siblings in *The Riveras* on NBC Universo. Chiquis launched her music career in 2014, making her musical debut on international television at the Premios Juventud. Her 2015 memoir, *Forgiveness*, was an instant *New York Times* bestseller. Chiquis lives in Los Angeles, California.

SARAH KOUDOUZIAN is the CEO of BootyFit Workout, a celebrity personal trainer, and a philanthropist, with a bachelor's degree in kinesiology from California State University, Northridge, as well as a certification in nutrition. Whether she's working out with Chiquis, touring across the United States training Prince Royce, getting actress Emeraude Toubia red-carpet ready, preparing former Miss Universe Dayanara Torres for *Mira Quién Baila*, or training YouTuber Amy Serrano, Sarah believes that being fit is not about conforming to a specific look or size. It is about creating a healthy lifestyle. She currently resides in California. For more information, visit bootyfitworkout.com or YouTube.com /bootyfitworkout.